WI WATCHERS

The Beginners Guide to Weight Watchers Including a 30 day plan for rapid weight loss

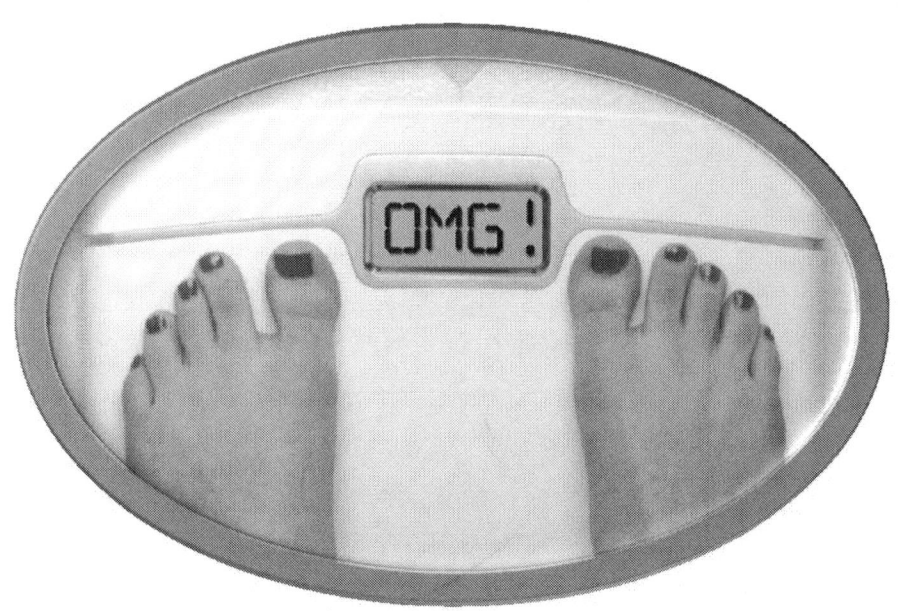

Michael Smith

@ Copyright 2018 by Michael Smith - All rights reserved.

This document is geared towards providing exact and reliable information in regards to the topic and issue covered. The publication is sold with the idea that the publisher is not required to render accounting, officially permitted, or otherwise, qualified services. If advice is necessary, legal or professional, a practiced individual in the profession should be ordered.

- From a Declaration of Principles which was accepted and approved equally by a Committee of the American Bar Association and a Committee of Publishers and Associations.

In no way is it legal to reproduce, duplicate, or transmit any part of this document in either electronic means or in printed format. Recording of this publication is strictly prohibited and any storage of this document is not allowed unless with written permission from the publisher. All rights reserved.

The information provided herein is stated to be truthful and consistent, in that any liability, in terms of inattention or otherwise, by any usage or abuse of any policies, processes, or directions contained within is the solitary and utter responsibility of the recipient reader. Under no circumstances will any legal responsibility or blame be held against the publisher for any reparation, damages, or monetary loss due to the information herein, either directly or indirectly.

Respective authors own all copyrights not held by the publisher.

The information herein is offered for informational purposes solely, and is universal as so. The presentation of the information is without contract or any type of guarantee assurance.

The trademarks that are used are without any consent, and the publication of the trademark is without permission or backing by the trademark owner. All trademarks and brands within this book are for clarifying purposes only and are the owned by the owners themselves, not affiliated with this document.

Table of Contents

Introduction 8
    What is the Weight Watchers Diet? 9
    Basics of the Weight Watchers Plan 12
    Why Choose Weight Watchers? 16
    What Foods Can I Eat? 19
    Getting Started with Weight Watchers 21
    What are the SmartPoints®? 22
    The Smart Points History 25
    The benefits of the Smart Points 27
    The negatives of Smart Points 28
    How do the Meetings Work? 30
    The Benefits of the Meetings 31
    Massive Health Benefits 35
    Fast Food And Eating Out 43
    How To Use Your Points 45
    Being Active Can Help 46
    The rules of working out 49
    What if I don't have time to work out? 51
    The benefits of working out 53
A 30 Day Meal Plan to Get You Started 57
Weight Watchers Breakfasts 64
    Pancakes – 6 SmartPoints® 65
    Healthy Morning Cookies – 2 SmartPoints® 66

Cinnamon Rolls—6 SmortPoints 67

Mushroom and Spinach Quiche – 3 SmartPoints® 68

Apple Muffin – 7 SmartPoints® 69

Potato and Cheese Casserole – 7 SmartPoints® 70

Crispy Apple Surprise – 11 SmartPoints® 71

Breakfast Jelly Pudding – 11 SmartPoints® 72

Pumpkin Muffins – 4 SmartPoints® 73

Blackberry and Peach Smoothie – 9 SmartPoints® 74

Morning Burritos – 9 SmartPoints® 74

Breakfast Souffle – 3 SmartPoints® 76

Breakfast Bars – 6 SmartPoints® 77

French Toast – 3 SmartPoints® 78

Cheese and Ham Omelet – 6 SmartPoints® 78

Spiced Honey Cake – 7 SmartPoints® 79

Blueberry Muffins – 5 SmartPoints® 81

Yogurt Fluff – 2 SmartPoints® 82

Weight Watchers Lunches 83

Creamy Pesto Pasta – 7 SmartPoints® 84

BBQ Pork Sandwich – 5 SmartPoints® 85

Italian Chicken – 5 SmartPoints® 86

Baked Tortellini – 6 SmartPoints® 87

Cheesy Mushrooms – 2 SmartPoints® 89

Baked Burrito – 6 SmartPoints® 90

Italian Bread with Tuna Salad – 10 SmartPoints® 91

Turkey and Cheese Sandwich – 10 SmartPoints® 92
Veggie Soup – 1 SmartPoint 93
Cheeseburger Soup – 7 SmartPoints® 94
Pasta Veggies – 5 SmartPoints® 95
Bacon Wrap – 8 SmartPoints® 96
Baked Fish – 5 SmartPoints® 97
Beef Ziti Bake – 7 SmartPoints® 98
Chicken Salad – 4 SmartPoints® 99
Egg Salad – 4 SmartPoints® 100
Beef Burgers – 4 SmartPoints® 101

Dinners on Weight Watchers For The Whole Family 102
Cheesy Chicken Chops == 3 Smart Points 102
Jalapeno Chicken – 5 SmartPoints® 103
Cilantro Lime Shrimp – 3 SmartPoints® 104
Spinach and Chicken Crescents == 4 SmartPoints® . 105
Steak and Mashed Potatoes – 8 SmartPoints® 105
Honey Salmon – 4 SmartPoints® 106
Veggie Pork Chops – 6 SmartPoints® 107
Mexican Casserole – 8 SmartPoints® 108
Chicken Thai Wrap – 2 SmartPoints® 109
Pita Bread Pizza – 9 SmartPoints® 110
Potato Soup – 4 SmartPoints® 111
Roast Beef with Veggies – 8 SmartPoints® 112
Mushroom Steak – 5 SmartPoints® 112

Cheese and Tuna Sandwich – 10 SmartPoints® 114

Cola Chicken – 5 SmartPoints® 115

Beef Chili – 4 SmartPoints® 116

Vegetable Quesadilla – 9 SmartPoints® 117

Baked Chicken – 10 SmartPoints® 118

Chicken and Dumplings – 9 SmartPoints® 118

Conclusion 120

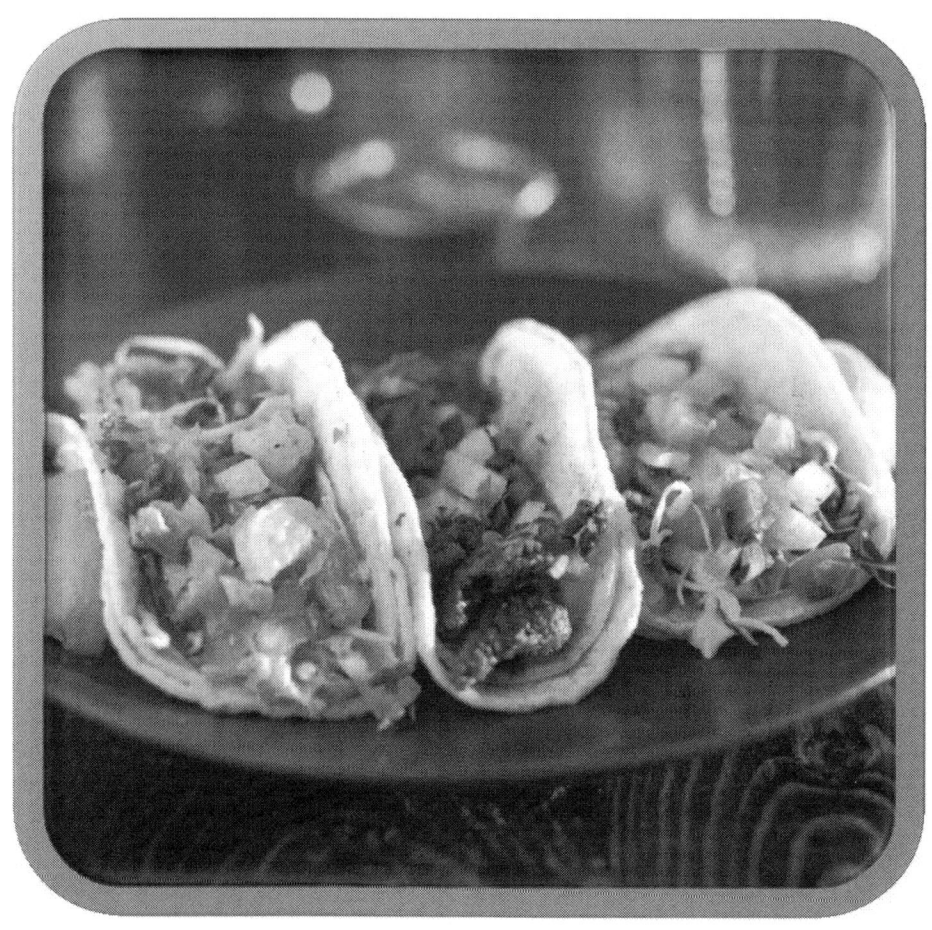

Introduction

When it comes to picking out the right diet plan that you are going to use, there are a lot of options that you can choose from. All of them are going to offer advice and suggestions on what you are able to do to lose weight, but many of them are unsafe, offer bad advice, and are just too hard to follow for the long term.

This guidebook is going to spend some time talking about the Weight Watchers plan, a plan that is going to help you to lose weight and get in better health for your whole life and not just for a few weeks. We are going to explore how to make this diet plan work the best for your needs.

When you are first looking to lose weight or get in better health than you were before, you will find that there are a lot of different weight loss plans that you are able to follow. Some are going to ask you to limit the types of certain foods that you are allowed to eat, some will limit the times that you are allowed to eat during the day, and some can be really unhealthy and unsafe (even if they do drop some of the pounds in the beginning). All of this information can be hard to sift through and you may feel worried that you are not able to find the right diet plan with the right rules that will work for you.

Most Americans are living an unhealthy lifestyle and because of this, there are a ton of weight loss and diet programs out there. Americans are eating more calories than ever, most of which are going to be full of saturated fats, sugars, and other things that are bad on the body. Add to this that most of these same people are going to live a sedentary lifestyle that includes sitting in front of the desk all of the time and then going home and just watching television all of the time. All of this is going to add together in order to make you feel unhealthy and gain a lot of weight in the process.

What is the Weight Watchers Diet?

Weight Watchers is one of the best diet plans that you can choose. It is not going to be as restrictive as some of the other diet plans that are out there. You are not going to have to pick whether you are allowed to eat grains or eating some fats in your diet. You will get to pick out the foods that you would like to eat, but you will be limited rather on the amount of points, known as SmartPoints® in this program, that you are allowed to eat each day. This makes it a little bit healthier to follow because you will be able to choose a lot of healthy and tasty foods, you won't be stuck eating foods that are unhealthy and bad for the body or having to feel like you are deprived all the time.

Let's take a look at this program a bit more. The idea behind Weight Watchers is to make you more conscious about the food choices that you are making. Many diet plans tell you to avoid this or that and then concentrate too much on the amount of calories that you are consuming. As long as you are staying in this calorie count, they promise that you are going to lose weight. The issue with this is that it isn't always about the amount of calories that you are eating as it is about the type of calories that you eat. 100 calories of fruit are much different than a 100 calories of a cookie and this is kind of how the Weight Watchers diet is going to focus on.

With the diet, you are going to be given a set amount of SmartPoints® that you are allowed to have each day and then you are able to have a few more during the week for when you want a cheat day or to eat out every once in a while. The amount of points that you are allowed will be based on your own personal profile. Depending on your height, current weight, and how much you would like to lose, you will be given an amount of SmartPoints® that you are able to use up each week.

Note: The SmartPoints® have been changed a bit in the last few years. In the past, participants were able to workout each day and then add in some more of the points each day. This started to develop an unhealthy relationship between working out and the foods that the participants were eating. While exercise is an important part of this whole process and can help you to keep healthy, it is not a good idea to think about food being the reward for the exercise that you do each day.

The foods that are healthier for you, such as healthy carbs, protein, and fruits and vegetables are going to be given fewer points, meaning that you are able to eat more of them. On the other hand, the foods that are considered bad, the ones that are full of sugars, saturated fats, and other bad things are going to have a higher point value for each serving. You are not forbidden from eating certain foods during this diet plan, but when you are faced on the choice of eating all your calories for the day in two pieces of cake or getting a few balanced meals, you are more likely to choose the latter.

One of the reasons that Weight Watchers is so much more effective than you will find with some of the other diet plans is because of the meetings. Not only are you going to concentrate on eating the right foods and trying to get in a bit more exercise and activity to your daily routine, you will also need to attend meetings. These meetings are where you will be held accountable for your weight loss and the choices that you make. You will have a private weigh-in each time that you go, feel encouraged to keep meeting your goals, and even hear stories and get advice on how to keep going.

Most people find that while these meetings are a bit intimidating in the beginning, they are going to make a big difference in the amount of weight that you will lose overall. You will be able to ask your questions, get advice, and find out whether you are staying on track of the diet plan or not.

In addition to eating the right kinds of foods, you will need to pay attention to the amount of exercise that you are getting each day. While you will not be able to get more points for food any longer when your workout, you will still need to add in some more exercise in order to work out the heart, lose more weight, and feel even better. Make sure to add in at least 30 minutes of moderate exercise most days of the week and you are going to feel so much better than you did in the past.

Basics of the Weight Watchers Plan

Weight Watchers is one of the best weight loss programs you can get on. It allows you to lose a lot of weight in a safe and effective way. While some of the other diet plans make a lot of promises along the way, most of them are hard to keep up or leave you feeling deprived for the long term. When it comes to Weight Watchers, you are able to maintain it because it is so easy and simple to follow. You can live life while on this diet, still having a few treats and getting to eat out when you would like, but you just have to be a bit smarter about the choices that you make when it comes to the foods that you eat.

The Weight Watchers program is based on a points system. When you attend our first meeting or sign up online, you will be able to learn how many points you are allowed to have during the day. The points that you get will vary based on how much you want to lose, and some other factors including weight, age, height, and activity level. The point levels will change during your journey to help you adjust to any weight loss that you have and ensures that you will continue to see results along the way.

These points are going to really help you along the way. They don't tell you exactly what you have to eat, but they will help you to pick the right choices. Foods that are high in protein and lots of good nutrients, such as vegetables, fruits, and lean meats, will be lower in points. This means that you would be able to eat more of them before you met your point values. Options that are high in bad fats, carbs, and sugars are going to be higher in points. This means that you would be able to eat fewer of them before reaching your point allowance.

Now, you are able to have a treat on occasion if you would like, but you just need to be smart about how you are doing with it. Plus, if you are allowed to have a lot of one type of food when you are hungry and not so much of another, you are probably more likely to pick the food that is healthier so that you can eat a little bit more.

You can even use these points when you go out to eat. You will be able to learn how to calculate the points for what you would like toe at when you go out (and since the Weight Watchers plan is so prevalent, many restaurants will include the points totals for you on the menu), and then you can make smart choices that will help you to keep losing the weight, even when you want to go out and have some fun.

The idea behind the Weight Watchers plan is to not deprive you, but to just help you to make some healthier choices. This diet plan realizes that there are days when things are tough and you would like to eat something that is a little sweet or bad for you. It understands that there are times you want to go out and celebrate with friends and have some fun. There are no rules against doing these things you just need to learn how to use your points correctly so that you can really see the results.

In addition to being able to use the SmartPoints® to stay on track with your weight loss, you will find that the meetings are also helpful. These are available in many areas around the country, but if you aren't able to make the meeting times in your area or you are too far away from one, you can also do the meetings online. This is where you will meet others who are on the same journey as you, ask some of the questions that you have, get lots of advice, and even do your weigh-ins to see how you are doing. Don't worry about having to share your weight with anyone else. First this is a supportive community of people ho are on the same journey as you are and second, you will be able to do the weigh-ins in private so you won't have to worry about anyone else knowing how well you are doing or if you fell behind on a week.

It is a really good idea to go to the meetings as often as you can. These help to hold you accountable and result in people on this plan losing a lot more weight than if they did it all on their own without the meetings. You are also going to meet a lot of amazing people who are trying to lose weight as well, or who already lost weight with this program, and they can give you inspiration to keep on working hard for the results that you want.

You should also make sure that you are getting in plenty of exercise during the week. This is a part that a lot of people miss out on sometimes, but it is so important for the overall health of your heart and body. While Weight Watchers has made some changes in terms of the relationship between their points and exercise in order to foster a healthier relationship between the two, it is still important to get some movement in each day to make the muscles and heart stronger. Try to do a combination of aerobics, weight lifting, and stretching on most days of the week to really help out with our weight loss goals.

There are also many health benefits that you can enjoy when using the Weight Watchers system. You will first notice that it helps you to lose a lot of weight. Since you are reducing a lot of the calories that you consume each day, you will be able to enjoy a lot of weight loss. Plus, your body is getting in so many good nutrients that it will feel like it is filled up and more energized than you did on your old diet plan.

You may also notice that your heart health is getting better than before. The healthy foods that you are eating, and the ones that you get rid of, will help to nourish the heart, limit high blood pressure, and can even take care of some of that cholesterol that is causing some issues. You may also notice that while you are on the Weight Watchers plan, you are eating fewer sugars so it is easier to lower your bad blood sugars and maybe even take care of some of those issues that come with diabetes.

Other benefits that you may notice while being on this simple diet plan includes more energy, better mood because your mind feels like it is opened up and ready to take on the day, lower joint pain from all that acidic food you are eating and so much more. There is just so much that you will be able to see improved when you are on the Weight Watchers plan that it is worth your time to give this diet plan a try.

If you are looking for a new diet plan and you are tired of all the hard work and impossible tasks that are placed out in some of your other diet plans of the past, it may be time to try out the Weight Watchers diet plan. This one is simple to use and will be able to help you get the results that you want without being impossible. While other diet plans have you eat things that are unhealthy or limit you so much that you are bound to fail at some point, Weight Watchers is meant for your daily life.

This diet plan allows you to have some of the snacks and some of the sweets that you crave, as long as you are careful about how you eat for the majority of the time. This diet realizes that you may have tough days or those days that you want to go out and celebrate, and it makes sure that you are getting the right nutrition while still eating out and having fun on occasion.

It also provides you with a support group to get through the good and the tough times when they come up. There is just so much to love about this particular diet plan and you are going to love how easy it is to get on and follow!

Why Choose Weight Watchers?

There are a lot of great diet plans that you can choose to go with. Some are going to choose to have you limit your carb intake while others are going to limit the fats. Some are healthy while others are going to be hard to maintain because they are so hard on the body. Weight Watchers is a bit different than all of these because you get some options. Some of the reasons that you should choose to go with Weight Watchers instead of another weight loss program includes:

- Lose more weight—overall, people who go on a program similar to Weight Watchers are able to lose more weight than with other options. This is because it is flexible to follow and you have that motivation and support going to the meetings each week.
- Flexibility—there is a lot of flexibility that comes with being on Weight Watchers. You get to enjoy the ability to pick the foods that you want to consume, when you want to eat them, and even how much based on the amount of points that you are going with. You can also pick your activity levels, your meetings, whether to have the meetings in person or online and so much more! This makes it easier for everyone to find the path on this plan that works best for them.
- Lifestyle change—weight watchers is not just about losing weight. It is about making changes in your whole lifestyle that will result in healthy weight loss. You are going to learn how to eat foods that are healthier and full of nutrition while getting rid of the foods that are causing

weight gain and health issues. You are going to learn how important activity is in your life and star to implement it in more. You will work on getting healthier stress levels and sleeping as well.
- Eat the foods you like—you are the one in charge of the foods that you eat on this diet plan, so you can eat some of your favorites as well. While you do need to make some healthier choices when it comes to staying within your points, there is still the option of having some of your favorite meals on occasion.
- Ability to fit it into your daily life—it is possible to fit this diet plan into your daily life. You are able to eat real foods, foods that taste good, and will fill you up. You can choose to workout each day or do normal activities, such as chores, around the house, without having to spend hours at the gym each day. The foods can be your normal favorites as long as you are careful about not eating too much.
- You can eat out—when you are on this plan, you are allowed to eat out. While you shouldn't do this each day, eating out every once in a while is not a bit sin of this diet plan. It realizes that there are times you will go out with friends and family and realizing that you can go out as long as you make the right decisions for the rest of the day and don't overdo it with eating at the restaurant, you will be fine without ruining all your hard work.

- People to help you along the way—there are weekly meetings that you can attend that will help you to stay on your plan. You can meet with others who will motivate you along your journey and will help you any time that things get stuff or you need some help. It is hard to find this kind of motivation on the other diet plans that you pick.

There is no diet plan that is the same as Weight Watchers for all the flexibility and support that you are going to get along the way. If you have been trying to lose weight in the past and are ready to take that step to seeing a lot of success finally, make sure to check out Weight Watchers and see how it can work for you.

What Foods Can I Eat?

One of the first questions that people are going to have when they get on the Weight Watchers program is what foods they are allowed to eat. You want to have a good idea of the foods that are allowed and the ones that aren't allowed so that you can plan accordingly when making your meals or going to the grocery store. When it comes to the Weight Watchers plan, you will see that you are not really limited on the types of food that you are allowed to eat, although you are certainly going to be guided to pick ones that are healthier. Weight Watchers understands that staying on a diet can be tough and if you are always told that you can't have something or you will lose all that hard work, you are going to crave that thing all the more. While you should concentrate on eating mostly healthy foods and staying in your allotted points, there is some freedom to have something a little "bad" for you on occasion and this is even added into the points that you can have each week.

This is not an invitation to eat as many of the bad things that you want each week and still hope to lose weight. There are a few extra points that are added to your weekly total, but they are not enough for you to go crazy with. They are there to allow you to get the amount of calories that you need to stay healthy and for a little bit of treat when you just can't fight the cravings.

While there aren't really any limits on the foods that you are able to eat, you do need to stick with the points that are given to you at the meeting. Keep in mind that as you lose weight these point amounts are going to go down a bit so that you are able to keep on losing weight. The beauty of these points is that they are going to help you to make the healthy choices, so you end up eating fewer calories, as well as better foods, in the long run.

Think of it this way, would you like to waste all of those points that you have for the day on a big coffee at Starbucks, or would it be better to have three nice meals with a lean protein, some milk, and some vegetables along with a nice snack of fruits? In most cases, you are going to go for the latter option because it helps you to feel full, gives your body the right nutrition, and can make you feel better. Of course, you are allowed to have that dessert on occasion, but you will learn that it isn't always worth it to give into the cravings and will instead pick to go with the healthier foods.

Getting Started with Weight Watchers

It is actually pretty simple to get started with Weight Watchers. You will start out by finding a meeting that is in your area; if you find that the meetings are not in your area or you just aren't able to make the times that are in your area, you can also sign up for the meetings online as well. Even if you do want to go to the meetings in person most of the time, you may find that there are some great online tools that you are able to use to help you stay on track in between some of your meetings.

When you find a local Weight Watchers meeting, you are going to find that you are getting into a group that has a lot of great individuals. All of these people have either gone on their weight loss journey or are working on it at that time and all of them are on the Weight Watchers program. This can make it easier to connect to the people who are working towards the same goals as you and they will help you to stay on track, live a healthier lifestyle, and get the results that you want.

Some people are scared about doing these meetings, but there is nothing to worry about. They are a lot of fun, you get to meet new people and share stories, you get the encouragement that you need to feel amazing, and all of your results are going to be private so no one else will know!

Overall, this is one of the best diet plans that most people will choose to go with. it allows you to eat a lot of the foods that you enjoy while getting a few of those cheat days on occasion without having to worry about it all the time. While it will take some adjusting to look at the foods that you are eating based on how many points they are worth, the Weight Watchers plan can make it easier than ever to eat right, pick the foods that are healthier, and lose that weight, while gaining that good health, that you have been looking for.

Following Weight Watchers is a great option that is going to help you to not only lose weight, but also to take care of the other unhealthy parts of your diet. You are going to love not only that the inches are coming off, but that you are able to get more energy, that you feel better, and that your lifestyle in general is just better than before.

As this chapter and the rest of the guidebook talks about, Weight Watchers is a lifestyle change, one that you are able to maintain for the long term without having to starve yourself or feel miserable all the time. With the help of the points and meetings, you will find that Weight Watchers is not a fad and that you can make it work for you!

What are the SmartPoints®

With Weight Watchers, you are not necessarily kicking out any of the food groups, you are just becoming more conscious about the food decisions that you make.

This diet plan realizes that you are going to want that piece of cake or that cookies on occasion and telling you that you are not allowed to have it will simply make the situation worse. The idea behind Weight Watchers is that you are allowed to have some of these snacks and goodies, as long as you fit it properly within your diet.

When you go on Weight Watchers, you are going to be given a points system. This is to help you to make decisions based on your current weight and how much you would like to use in the process. These are the amount of points that you are able to use up during the day and can help you to make healthier food choices. Each food that you pick will have a certain point value and the goal is to stay within the points each day.

Now as mentioned, you are allowed to eat some of those sweets, but if you are at the end of the day and have only five points left, you may reach for an apple rather than going for that piece of cake that is worth 15 and would put you over your point goal.

You get to decide how to use the points and there are lots of handbooks that will help you to see how many points each of your food choices are. If you do want that piece of cake in the day (perhaps you know you are heading to a birthday party), you will be able to budget ahead of time to pick out wholesome and healthy foods that will keep you within your points allowance without missing out on nutrition.

You will need to be careful about these points. Some people get too excited about losing weight and will try to limit their calories too much. This may seem like a good idea; they assume that if they only use half their calories each day, they will lose the weight faster. But the issue here is that you may be cutting calories, but you are also cutting out healthy nutrition that the body really needs. You need to be careful about doing this.

There may be days when you aren't as hungry or you are too busy to eat as much as you should and your points values will be a bit lower. You don't need to force yourself to eat on these days. But you should aim to get close to your point totals each day so that you are giving your body adequate nutrition and calories to keep functioning.

These points are going to be really important when it comes to the foods that you are allowed to eat on this diet plan. Rather than focusing on the calories that you are consuming, you are going to focus on the points. These points are based on the macro and micro nutrients that are inside of the food that you plan to eat during the day.

When the food has a lot of good macro and micro nutrients like protein, good carbs, and healthy vitamins, you are going to see that they contain a smaller amount of points and you are able to eat more of them throughout the day with your diet.

On the other hand, if the items are mostly calories, sugars, and saturated fats, they are going to rank higher when it comes to the points that you are able to use. The idea behind this is that you are encouraged to eat more of the healthier foods while ditching some of the bad foods, although some of these bad foods are allowed on occasion when you are on the diet plan.

These points are going to allow you to make the best decisions when it is time to pick out the foods that you want to enjoy. You are going to be able to enjoy some of the treats on occasion when you want, but overall, you will choose to go out and eat the healthier foods because they fill you up more, you can eat more of them without having to use up all of your points, and they will taste so amazing in the process!

The Smart Points History

During 2016, Weight Watchers made some changes to their points system. They had received some criticism that their program was too much about the points and not enough about the nutritional content of the foods people were picking.

People could easily miss out on the healthy nutrients that they needed or pick foods that were high in sugars and saturated fats and still stick within the guidelines that were set out with Weight Watchers. This is why Weight

Watchers came out with the new "Smart Points" and the "Beyond the Scale" program in 2016.

The Smart Points have made it easier to count out your points and they are going to push you towards foods that are healthier and more nutritious. This has a lot of great benefits including helping you to feel better, lose weight, and gain more energy at the same time. The food items that may have had lower points totals before, such as those with sugar and saturated fats, now have higher point values. Protein sources and fresh produce will have lower points values.

You are still in charge of the foods that you would like to eat, but the points are going to encourage you to pick foods that are healthier so that you are able to stay within your points value. The new point system is going to reward you for eating less saturated fat and less sugar while eating more protein in your diet.

The Activity Points have now been replaced with the FitPoints within Weight Watchers and they are going to be calculated out based on the activities that you are doing each week. The activities can range from planned exercises to just doing chores around the house during the day.

In addition to your normal points values that you are given, the original points in Weight Watchers would give you an extra 49 that you are able to use in the way that you wanted. These can be nice for that one cheat day or when you are just feeling really hungry on one of your days. The

Smart Points still have these extra calories, but they are going to be adjusted based on the individual person and may include factors like age, gender, your goals for weight loss, and even your activity levels.

The benefits of the Smart Points

There are a lot of benefits that come from using Smart Points for your weight loss goals and this is part of why the Weight Watchers system is so popular. Some of the benefits of going with this system includes:

- The Smart Points help to keep you to pick healthier foods that are good for you. You will be docked any time that you choose foods that are full of sugars and saturated fats while those who chose healthier options would be set.
- The Smart Points got rid of the unhealthy notion that if you exercise more, you can eat more. Most people overestimate their activity level so this led to them having issues with weight loss, plus they were still eating the unhealthy foods in the process. with the Smart Points, you will not be able to add in more points when you exercise more, so you will separate out the activity that you do from the foods that you eat.
- These Smart Points are going to focus more on having a healthier lifestyle. While weight loss is a part of this, you are going to find that it is more about the healthier lifestyle rather than just

counting calories and worrying yourself sick over everything that you eat.

The negatives of Smart Points

While there are a lot of positives that you will be able to get from using the points system from Weight Watchers, there are a few people who have voiced concerns over the new Smart Points, especially those who were used to the old system with Weight Watchers. Some of the complaints that have come up in regards to these points include:

- Some people are worried that these points are making it more difficult to pick out foods. There isn't as much flexibility and freedom in the points. If you were used to the old Points Plus system, you may really notice this.
- There are a lot of restrictions. The restrictions for eating things like cake and cookies on the new Smart Points program is so high, that many will want to give up on the whole program. While it is an adjustment, most people who seriously wanting to lose weight will not see an issue with these and will stay on the plan.

When you join Weight Watchers, you will be able to work with a coach, whether you work online or you go in person to the meetings. They will be able to fill out your profile to figure out how much you weight, how much you want to lose, how tall you are, your age, and other things that will influence your health and how much weight you can loose on the system. Things like being older in age or wanting to lose more weight will really slow down the metabolism and will need to be taken into consideration.

With this information, your coach will be able to determine how many points are a good place for you to start and will give you suggestions on staying healthy and making the right meal choices. Over time, you will be able to meet with your coach again and adjust the values based on whether you need to lose more weight, are losing too much weight, or just want to maintain the weight loss that you have already accomplished.

Either way, the points value system in Weight Watchers is a great way to get started on the system and will ensure that you are picking out the best foods for your body to stay healthy, get more energy, and to even lose some weight in the process. Keep in mind that when you get started on this whole program, you will lose weight in most cases, but the process is more about changing out the unhealthy aspects of your lifestyle rather than losing the weight.

Most of the other programs that you are going to choose will not work on this points system. They are going to just tell you the foods that you are allowed to eat and the ones that you should avoid. They will tell you how many calories that you should have and will place so many restrictions on you that it is too hard to keep up with during the daily life that you are living.

On the other hand, when you are using the SmartPoints® system, you aren't going to be so limited. You are able to take care of your own decisions when picking out foods. You can mix things up a bit and have a wide variety of foods rather than being stuck with just a few meals that fit in with the diet plan. When you are ready to try out something that is going to help you to lose weight while still maintaining some of your own individuality and without ruining your whole day, Weight Watchers is the best option for your weight loss goals.

There are some people who like using the SmartPoints® to help them to limit the bad foods and eat the good foods that will actually help them to lose the weight that they want. Others feel like this is too easy for some people and that it isn't really helping them to concentrate on the right foods in the right way since you are still allowed to eat some of the foods that are bad for you. Either way, this is one of the most popular diet plans on the market and many people have seen a lot of results when it comes to their health and weight loss goals with Weight Watchers.

How do the Meetings Work?

When you are first getting started with Weight Watchers, you probably hear about the meetings. This is something that many of the members participate in and they will ask you to come along with them to check out the meetings.

For some people, the meetings can be a bit intimidating. They are worried about having to talk too much at the meetings or that someone is going to make fun of them if they have trouble losing weight.

The meetings are not that scary (the weigh ins are confidential so you don't have to worry about this part), and you are going to be able to see a lot of results with them. The meetings are meant to help you to stay accountable for the work that you should be accomplishing. Many people are able to do a better job with losing weight and gaining a healthier lifestyle when they are able to have someone hold them accountable.

Let's take a look at some of the aspects that come with the Weight Watchers meetings and why you should consider joining one of these meetings each week, whether you choose to go with the in person meetings are the online meetings for your needs.

The Benefits of the Meetings

One of the aspects that you will learn about when you join Weight Watchers is that there are meetings that you should attend. Traditionally these were in person meetings where you could meet with others, weigh yourself, get advice and support, and more. But with the busy times that many people have, Weigh Watchers has expanded to have online meetings for those who don't live near an in person meeting, those who are too busy for the meetings, or those who are just more comfortable doing it on their own.

There have been a lot of studies that Weigh Watchers is one of the few programs for weight loss that actually has long term results. One of the factors that is contributing to this is the fact that there are in person meetings while other diet plans do not have these. Sure, you are going to have to spend time keeping track of your own progress, but when you have to go to regular meetings and be held accountable for your success, it is easier to lose some that weight.

Over 40 years ago, this program was started as just an idea to gather some women to a weekly meeting in order to help each other to lose some weight. These meetings were great because not only did you get a chance to meet with others and socialize, you also got to be held accountable while receiving motivation and some educational materials that would help you to meet your goals.

These meetings were one of the best places to learn more about the points systems, to ask your questions, and to even hear how you can make healthier meal choices. There are many communities that have these meetings so it is often easy to find one that is near your home or you can use the Weight Watchers online program to help out as well.

The overall purpose of these meetings is to help you out on your weight loss journey. The overall purpose was to build up the knowledge that you have about weight loss and it gives you some of the tools that you need to lose weight as well as to change your lifestyle so that you can keep the weight off. When each meeting is done, you are going to also receive some information that will help you to stick with your plans.

Each of the meetings for Weight Watchers is run by a Meeting Leader. The nice thing about these leaders is that they have been a member of Weight Watchers, and many of them have gone through the program themselves in order to lose weight. This means that they have the knowledge to help you lose your weight and to work with the program well. You will also receive some insights from them on how to stay on the journey and to develop a new healthy relationship with the food that you are eating.

At each of the meetings that you go to, you will have a weigh in. this is going to be private so you won't have to worry about others learning about your weight. The weight loss weigh in is a good way to monitor how your progress is going and can ensure hat you are staying accountable for any losses and gains that you have during the week. The weigh in is going to be done either by the receptionist or by the meeting leader.

After the weigh ins, the leader will spend some time discussing a new topic. These can range from health, weight loss, fitness, eating, and other topics that will help you on your journey. You do not need to join in on the discussion at all, but it is common for some of the other members to share their stories as well as some advice with others in the group.

This is a great time to meet others in your community who are working towards the same goals as you. There is no judgment here, just the hope of living a happier and healthier life. you are able to meet new people, discuss issues that are bothering you in regards to weight loss, and to get the support that you are looking for.

Weight Watchers has slowly moved to the online community as well. Even if you go to the in person meetings, some of the members will use online tools from Weight Watchers to help manage their plan and stay on track between meetings, especially if they need to miss a meeting along the way because things get busy.

Most communities are going to have a variety of times and days when you will be able to attend the meetings, so this makes it easier to fit into your schedule. With that being said, you can choose to go with the online option if you happen to be too busy for these meetings or you live in one of the areas where there are no meetings nearby.

You will do a lot of the same things as the in person meetings, including working with a weigh in, receiving new information for your plan, and you can even join forums to talk to others about their weight loss journey on the plan.

As you can see, the meetings in Weight Watchers are not all that scary. No one else is going to know how much weight you are losing or gaining in the process and you will be able to meet with some others in your area and discuss important weight loss and health topics along the way. This is really an important step when it comes to losing weight with this plan because it is going to help you to be held accountable.

Even if you are nervous about going for the first time, you can consider bringing along a friend or someone else that you know to make things easier. It isn't going to take you long though to realize how great a lot of the people are in these meetings and how they are going to have your back, and offer a lot of support at every stage of the journey with weight loss and good health and you will find that soon you will enjoy going to these meetings, even if you were a little nervous in the beginning.

If you are still worried about going to the meetings, see if you can find someone to go with you the first few times. There are also online meetings that you can go with to make it easier and to fit around your own personal schedule.

Massive Health Benefits

Any time that you go on a new diet plan, one that is healthy and is going to help you to lose weight, you are going to see quite a few health benefits. Gaining weight and following a diet and lifestyle plan that is not all that healthy is going to start wearing you down and can make you feel low on energy, have heart and blood pressure trouble, and can even add to your issues with diabetes and more.

A healthy diet like what you will find with being on Weight Watchers is going to help to fix a lot of these problems and can get you in better health than ever before. Some of the health benefits that you are going to see when you choose to get on Weight Watchers includes:

Losing weight

One of the main reasons that people decide to go on the Weight Watchers plan is because they want to lose weight. They may have tried to lose weight in the past or they just started to notice that their weight and their health issues have gotten out of hand. Either way, the Weight Watchers plan is a great method to losing weight in a healthy way.

While Weigh Watchers is more about changing your lifestyle to be healthier, the weight loss is one of the side effects of their healthier lifestyle. You are adding more activity into your day, you are limiting the unhealthy foods, and you are making changes so that the foods you pick are healthy and wholesome. When all of this comes together, you are going to lose some weight on the plan.

Simply by losing some weight, you are going to be able to lose a lot of the health issues that you have been dealing with. you are going to gain more confidence, feel better, and look better in your clothes when you are able to follow this program properly rather than sticking with some of the bad eating and lifestyle choices that you have been enjoying.

Fight off diabetes

If you have a history of diabetes in your family or you are worried about being close to diabetic now, you will need to consider getting on a healthier diet. Diabetes is manageable, but it is tough and you could end up with a hose of other medical issues in the process.

All the unhealthy foods that you are eating is what is going to make diabetes a reality for you. All the sugars that you take in from cakes, candies, sodas, energy drinks and more are wreaking havoc on the body. In addition, many processed carbs are found in the American diet and these can cause some issues as well since they are converted into sugars within the bloodstream and raise insulin levels.

The Weight Watchers plan works to limit some of these bad foods. Of course you can have them on occasion, but they need to become the exception rather than the normal when you are eating. When you have a bit of sugar or some processed carbs in your die ton occasion, and it is coupled with other foods that are really healthy, you are not going to receive quite as many of the bad side effects.

Lower blood pressure

The traditional American diet is full of lots of saturated fats, sodium, and other things that are really bad on your blood pressure. The typical American is going to take in two to three times as much sodium as their body needs each day and this is going to wreak a lot of havoc on their blood pressure. Over time, the heart is going to have to work harder to get the blood through as the arteries get tighter and close together, leading to a disaster for the heart.

Changing up some of the foods that you consume can help to limit the sodium you are consuming and will add in a few good nutrients that can help to reverse the bad effects in your body.

More energy

Keeping up with our fast paced world can seem like an impossible task. You have to keep track of all your work at home, school, work, and all the other obligations and you may fall into bed at the end of the day and wonder how you were able to keep up with it all. Or you may be one of those people who start to droop a bit after lunch time and have to go out for a soda or an energy drink right in the middle of the day.

If this sounds like you, it is time to make some changes in your diet. You are eating foods that are high in calories, but are not giving you the right nutrition or the right vitamins to keep the body moving. Instead, you will receive a high of energy for a short while before coming crashing down and needing to either eat more to keep u the energy, or consume some high sugar products.

But with a healthy diet like Weight Watchers, you are able to eat foods that fill you up and provide you with energy that is going to last for hours, rather than a few minutes. These foods are lower in calories but really high in healthy nutrients that the body needs to stay healthy and to keep moving properly.

Consider swapping out that high carb lunch or the meal at the local restaurant with healthy food options like a lean protein source and fruits and vegetables and see how energized you are by the end of the day.

Get better sleep

Sleep is so important for your whole body. Sometimes when we stress out too much about the things that are going on around us and we will not take care of our bodies in the process. We will eat unhealthy foods avoid exercising, and sleep may be one of the last things that are on our minds. But without sleep, it is hard to lose weight, or even maintain your current weight, manage your stress, and keep your health in good working order.

With the help of the healthier lifestyle that you are going to learn how to use with Weight Watchers, you are going to find that it is easier than ever to get some better sleep. You are providing your body with all the good nutrition and exercise that it needs to stay healthy and this makes it so much easier to reduce your stress, and even turn off some of that inner noise that keeps you up, so that you are able to get the sleep that you need.

Lower stress

Who doesn't have a lot of stress going on around them? It seems that everything is so stressful all of the time. You want to be able to enjoy life, but taking care of kids, worrying about family, running to all those activities, and worrying about how work is going and all the bills can add a lot of stress to your daily life. Most people are dealing with an overabundance of stress in their lives and most of them have no idea how to deal with this stress in a healthy way.

While stress may seem like something normal and that you won't be able to get to go away, it is going to cause a lot of issues to your body. Stress can cause headaches, weight gain, bad moods, high blood pressure, and a whole host of other issues. When you learn how to deal with your stress and take care of your body, like you will learn to do with Weight Watchers, you will find that a lot of the health issues that you are dealing with.

Sometimes, changing the way that you live your life by making it healthier will make a big difference in your stress levels. There are many healthy foods that can help to alleviate your stress levels; eating unhealthy foods can often make your stress levels go through the roof.

Adding in some healthy exercise is going to release some great happy endorphins into the body that will make you feel good and will reduce the stress. This can all help you to get more sleep during the night so that you aren't feeling so stressed out for not getting enough sleep. By the time that you learn how to use the Weight Watchers program, you will find that your stress levels have gone way down.

Dealing with your levels of stress is an important part to staying as healthy as possible. Sure there is always going to be some stress that is going on around us in between taking care of kids, work, school, activities, and other obligations. But a healthy diet and some other skills for relaxation can make all the difference in helping you to lose the weight that you want.

Better immunity

Are you tired of feeling sick all of the time? If someone near you gets sick with anything, are you sure to be the next one in line who is feeling down and out? You may need to make some changes to your diet in order to help out with these illnesses and going on a diet like Weight Watchers is sure to help with these.

Those who eat a healthy diet that has a lot of healthy vitamins and minerals are less likely to get sick as much as others do. Your immunity is getting the protection that it needs to stay healthy and to fight off all those bacteria and viruses that are trying to attack your body.

So if you are tired of spending so much time in the doctors' office and you want to finally feel your best, you need to get on a diet similar to Weight Watchers and see how well all this healthy food can make you feel.

There are so many benefits that you are going to be able to get when you start working with Weight Watchers. You will be able to see changes in your whole life, not just in your weight loss the inches that you lose around your waist. It is worth your time to start checking out a healthier diet, like the one that is provided in Weight Watchers, so that you can start feeling better in no time.

When it is time to start taking better care of your health and you know that the best way to do this is through the diet that you are enjoying on a daily basis, you will want to give Weight Watchers a try. This is a simple diet plan that is easy to follow and still gives you freedom, while also giving you some of the extra tools that you need to really see the results that you are looking for.

These are just a few of the benefits that you are going to see when you choose to go on the Weight Watchers diet plan. It has all the healthy options that you need, helps you to learn how to pick the right foods for you, and make it easier than ever to see the results that you are looking for!

Don't be fooled by some of the other diet plans that are out there. They will promise to help you lose weight or improve your health, but you will find that they ask you to do things that are hard or really bad for your health in order to lose weight.

With Weight Watchers, you will get all the nutrients that your body needs so that you can lose weight in the way that is the healthiest for your body and mind.

Fast Food And Eating Out

When you are on a diet plan, it is tempting to want to go out to eat on occasion. You want to go out and celebrate something that is important, you are having a craving for that particular kind of food, or there is another reason why you want to eat outside of the home.

With some of the other diet plans that you may follow, you may have to bring your own food or request a lot of changes be made to the food that you eat because you just don't know how to make it work with your diet.

While there are a lot of nice things about Weight Watchers, one of the things that you are going to enjoy the most is that you will still be able to go out to eat and enjoy yourself. This diet plan realizes that life is hard, that special occasions do come up, and that no one wants to always miss out just because the are on a diet.

Weight Watchers is going to work a bit differently than you will find with other diet plans. You don't need to feel guilty about going out and it is allowed on occasion. As long as you learn how to budget out the points that you are using during the day and make more conscious choices so that you pick the ones that are right for you.

You are allowed to go out to eat and enjoy yourself on this diet plan, you just need to plan things out and make sure that you are going with options that are healthy, taste good, and won't make you go over your points.

You will also notice that eating out is easiest with Weight Watchers. Since this diet plan has been around for a long time, it is common to see that a lot of restaurants will provide the points values on their menus.

Even if the restaurant doesn't provide this right away, you may be able to ask about it and see what they have available. You can also go online to see what the options are for the restaurant that you want to visit and check to see if these meal options will align with what you have still available.

You can have a few choices here. If you know that you will be eating out later in the day, you can move around the points that you have available for that day so that more can go with the eating out. You can eat more fruits and vegetables to ensure that the points stay low but you feel full and happy until dinner time.

Or, you can choose to use some of the extra points that you have on your week and use those along with the points that you have leftover for the day to have a good time.

Let's take some time to look at how you can prepare for eating out on the Weight Watchers Diet!

How To Use Your Points

While it is allowed to eat out when you are on this diet plan, you still need to be careful to stay within the points that you have been allotted on this diet plan, if you would like to see the results. If you have enough points to eat out for that meal and you haven't used up all your extras, eating out is perfectly acceptable.

It is going to be important that you search through some of the options that are available to you beforehand so that you can realize how many points each meal is going to take up so that you are able to make the decisions for the meal that are right for you.

There are some times when you will go to a restaurant and have no idea how many points things are going to be. If you didn't know which restaurant you were going to visit before heading out, this can seem like a scary time when trying to pick out the right meals.

The trick here is to bring along the tools that will help you to figure out how many points the meals will be so that you can make informed decisions. There are a number of booklets and guides that you can use that make it easier than ever to follow this diet plan and will ensure that you stay on track even when eating out.

With a little bit of planning ahead of time and making sure to budget out your points enough so that you can visit your favorite restaurants, you will see that eating out doesn't have to be a pain or take you off your diet plan.

Being Active Can Help

In addition to being smart about the things that you eat on Weight Watchers, it is important to take some time to add in physical activity to your daily routine. This means that you need to get up and get some movement into your day, rather than just sitting at the desk.

While you are able to lose some weight simply by changing the eating patterns that you are in, especially if those eating patterns were really bad in the beginning, but if you want to see really amazing results, and improve your heart and muscle health, you need to get up and move each day.

Too many Americans spend their time at a computer or in another job that just requires them to sit there. They will go hours without moving, and then when they are done, they sit in a car to commute home or they sit on the couch and just watch their favorite show without getting up and moving much.

When they do this each day, they are letting the muscles get worn out and old, without the good muscle tone, they are letting the heart slow down and not get its exercise, and they are slowing down the metabolism.

All of this combined with the unhealthy diet choices of many Americans will make people sick. It is easy to add on the pounds when you eat whatever you want without regards to how it will affect your body and it is even easier to pack on the pounds when you barely get up and move around during the day.

Remember that Weight Watchers is not just about the foods that you eat, even though these are really important too. It is about making changes to the whole unhealthy lifestyle that got you in this current position. This means that you need to not only make some changes to the foods that you are eating, but you also need to consider making some changes to your activity levels.

Originally when Weight Watchers came out, you would be able to earn some extra points in your day if you did some exercise. This was meant to help encourage you to get out there and take that walk or do another program that you wanted during the day.

You could add points based on how hard and long you worked out and even some basic chores around the house could be added into the mix to make some more points.

While this did work for some people, it had some drawbacks of creating unhealthy thinking patterns between food and exercising. Most people would exercise so that they could eat two pieces of cake rather than one, which is not the purpose of adding on those points; you were supposed to pick healthier options that would make the muscles happy and healthy, rather than going with the unhealthy options that just added calories.

There was also the problem of people adding on too many points and overestimating the work that they did during the activity. It is hard to know exactly how many calories you are burning with a workout and some would overdo it and say that they could have way more points than they should. Even if they calculated out their calorie burn properly, they would end up eating too much of the bad foods and not enough of the good ones with these extra calories.

Since this fostered such an unhealthy relationship between exercise and food in the user, Weight Watchers has changed up their exercise recommendations to something that is a bit better for the user and can foster healthier relationships between food and working out.

You are no longer going to be able to get extra points when you work out, but this doesn't mean that working out is not a good idea when going with Weigh Watchers.

Instead, your points are going to be calculated based on your current activity levels and your goals on the plan. If you end up working out quite a bit and losing weight quickly, the leader may work with you to add on more points, but you will not be adding on the extra points all on your own.

You need to be able to pick out the healthy foods with lots of nutrition on your own to fuel your body even when you have a good workout.

The idea is that you should exercise because it is good for your body, rather than because you can get some extra points in order to cheat some more. Exercise is so good for the body, but often it doesn't require as many extra calories as we think it does.

Doing a short workout during the day may enhance our muscle strength and our heart muscles, but it is not really going to need more than a few extra calories and if you are smart about your food choices, you still won't feel deprived. So unless you are a serious exerciser who is at the gym all day running hard, the amount of extra food you will need while working out is going to be really small.

The rules of working out

With that being said, there are a few things that you can keep in mind when you are getting started on a new exercise routine. These are going to help you to get started and ensure that you are getting the right kind of workout for your needs.

First, the type of exercise that you choose is going to make a big difference. You need to be able to pick out a wide variety of workouts to target your whole body. Cardio is the first type and you should spend three or four days a week getting some of this into your routine because it elevates the heart rate and ensures that your heart is getting some of the care that it needs. Plus, it is really great for weight loss because you can burn a lot of calories in the process.

That doesn't mean that the other workout types aren't important. Weight lifting should be done a few times a week as well because it really tones those muscles.

When the muscles are toned, your metabolism is going to burn a lot faster during the day while doing normal activities. So while you may not burn as many calories during the actual workout part like you do with cardio, the metabolism benefits can be amazing with weight lifting. And you can't forget about stretching.

Take some time on your off days and do a bit of stretching, such as yoga or another technique. This can help to give the muscles a good relaxation time after working so hard during the week, makes them stronger and leaner. And prevent injury.

Now, when it comes to how long you should workout, this is going to vary. It is recommended that you workout for 45 to 60 minutes at least three times a week if you want to lose weight. Some people choose to workout five or six day at 30 minutes so that it is easier to fit into their schedule then spending hours on the workout.

If you are just starting out with your exercise program and it has been awhile since you worked out, it is best to start out slow. Ten minutes is better than nothing and you can build up from there. Never say that you don't have time for a workout; you can fit three or four ten minute sessions into the day and once you are done, you have completed a full workout.

Make sure that you add a lot of variety in the workouts that you choose. Mix up your stretching, cardio, and weight lifting days.

Try out a bunch of different activities, even ones that you never have done before. Mixing it up helps to work on different muscles groups, which helps with weight loss, and can make it easier to enjoy your workout.

What if I don't have time to work out?

Some people worry that they aren't going to have time to workout. They imagine having to spend hours at the gym in order to get the extra activity that you need to really see the results that you want. But with Weight Watchers, you don't need to spend all this time in the gym.

You simply need to spend a bit of time a few days a week working out, and then find other ways to sneak a bit of exercise into your routine. Some of the simple ways that you are able to add in more activity to your schedule includes:

- Get up every hour-rather than sitting at your desk all day long and never moving, consider getting up for at least two to five minutes every hour. Walk around the office, do some jumping jacks, and just move around a bit. With five minutes every hour for an eight-hour day, you will end up with forty-five minutes of exercise. You can bring this home with you too. During your favorite show, do some sit ups and pushups during commercial breaks and you can get an extra fifteen to twenty minutes every hour.

- Park further away—any time that you need to take your car, make sure that you park far away from the door. It may be just a few extra steps, but you do this a couple of times each day and it really adds up.

- Work out during your lunch—working out during your lunch break can be one of the best decisions for you to make. You can spend even twenty minutes of your lunch break and then enjoy a healthy meal for the rest of it. This won't take up too much of your time but can be a great way to walk around the office, or workout in the gym nearby without changing up your schedule too much.

- Take the stairs—if you work in an office that is up past the first floor, consider going up the stairs rather than the elevator. If the office is too far up to walk, start out with a few flights and then taking the elevator the rest of the way. You will be able to increase your endurance over time and can go up more flights of stairs.

- Learn chair exercises—if you aren't able to get up that often from your chair at work, learn a few simple exercises that will allow you to work out the body without moving as much.

- Add movements to chores—you can get all sweaty just from cleaning the house. Make your movement deliberate and add some things to them, and you are sure to get the added workout that you want while making the house look nice.

- Play at the park—take your children to the park (walk there if you are able to) and then play around at the park. Chase them, use the monkey bars, go down the slides, and more. You will be surprised at how much of a workout this can end up being for you.

There is always time to add more exercise to your day, you just need to get a bit creative in order to make this happen. Whether you get up from your chair more often or sneak in the workouts a few times during the day, you are sure to find the results that you want.

The benefits of working out

There are a lot of benefits that you are going to enjoy when it comes to working out. You will see a big difference in the way that your body feels and reacts, you will be able to reduce your stress levels, and your mood is going to start feeling better in no time.

Even ten minutes a day can make a big difference in how you feel overall. Some of the great benefits that you are going to be able to see when you start working out include:

- Better mood—on those days when you are just mad at everyone and grumpy, it is time to get a workout. Even if you are feeling sad and down, it is time to get up there and enjoy a good workout. Ten to fifteen minutes is all you need to make the mood feel better and if you are able to workout for longer, you will find that your body feels so much better and accomplished when it's done.

- Clearer mind—there is just something about working out that will clear out the mind and make it feel so much better. If you are feeling foggy or like you just can't get any more work done for the day, and it is only lunch time, consider getting out there and getting in a good workout.

- Healthier heart—your heart needs a workout as well. You want to use cardio at least a few times a day to help the heart get up there and really get stronger. Even if you have to start out slowly in the beginning, you will find that working that heart with some good exercises, such as walking, running, swimming, and biking, will help you to get that heart in shape.

- Faster weight loss—when you workout, you are burning up calories. And the more calories that you burn up, the easier it is to lose weight. Your metabolism is going to be faster so that it is able to eat up all that extra fat that is sitting in the body and you will be able to see some of those weight loss results faster than ever.

- Toned muscles—sitting on that couch is not helping your muscles be strong and healthy. Rather, it is making them get soft and weak and waste away. You don't have to just work on weight lifting either; stretching and cardio still get those muscles up and moving so that you can see more tone in your body. Plus, these toned muscles are going to help you to speed up the metabolism, which is healthy whether you want to lose weight or not.

- Leaves you wanting more—while getting started on an exercise program may seem tough in the beginning and you may want to go out and do anything else, you are going to grow to love it. If you can just stay consistent with the work for some time, you are going to see some amazing results in the process. For example, you will start to look forward t getting to the workout and seeing how many results that you can get. If you are someone who gets bored with the workout, just have a plan to change it up every few months or so and you will be fine.

While many people dread working out and putting in all that effort, there really is a lot of good that can come from working out on a regular basis. Give it a chance along with the other pars of your Weight Watchers plan and see just how much it can change your results.

When you are first getting started with working out, you will find that it is really hard to get into a workout program. You will not want to get up there and do your workout, but over time, you are going to see how important it is to your health.

When you are able to see the great results, see how much you feel better, and see the boost in your mood, you are soon going to want to start working out.

You don't have to spend all day in the gym in order to see the results that you want with Weight Watchers. Just a little bit of activity each day to get the heart and muscles working strong is enough to make you feel amazing in no time.

A 30 Day Meal Plan to Get You Started

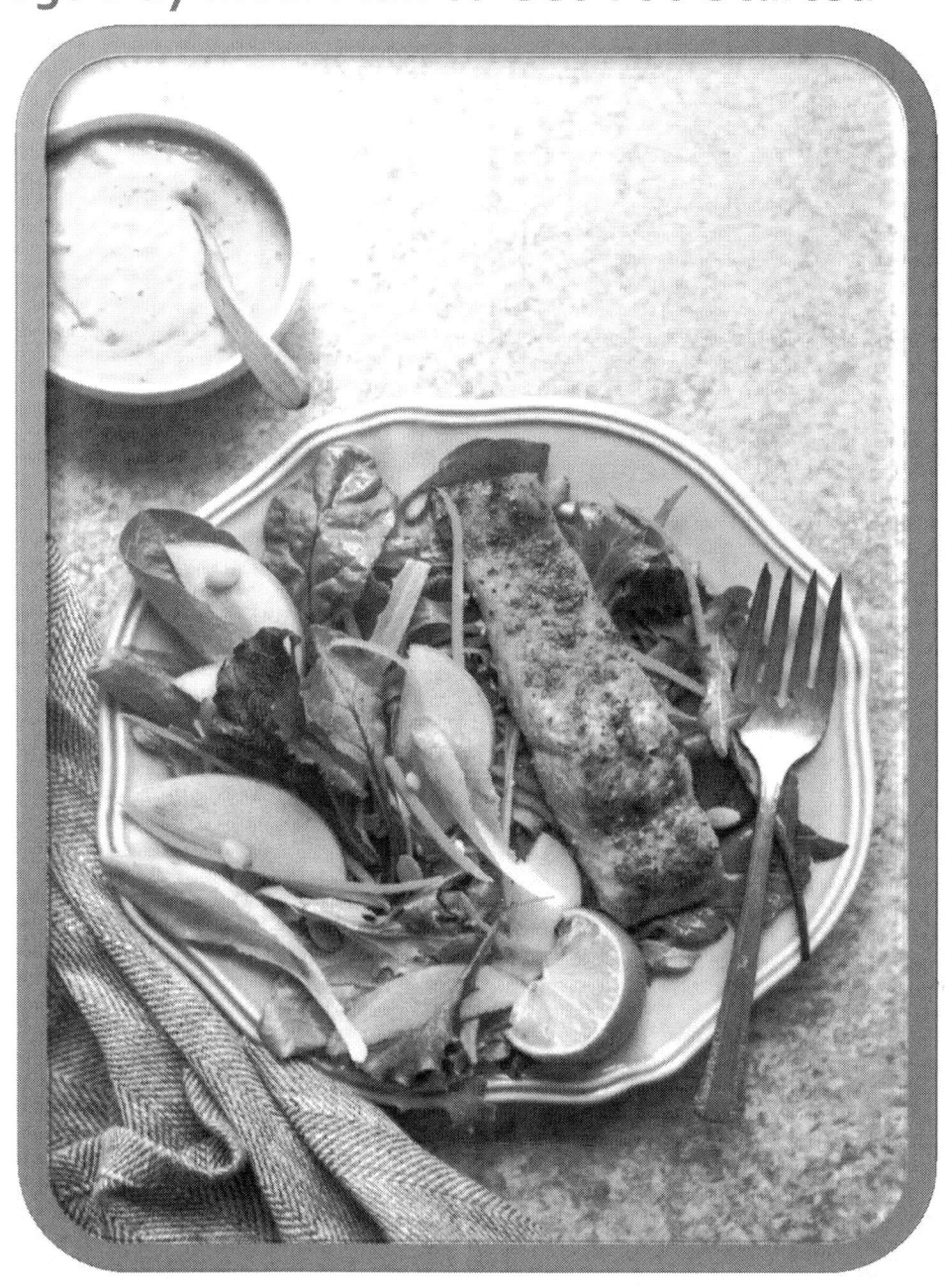

Sometimes one of the hardest things that you will need to do when it comes to getting started on a new meal plan is figure out what meals you would like to cook. There are so many meals out there, but learning which ones belong to your new diet plan and will not make you go over our daily limit can be kind of intimidating in the beginning.

In this chapter, we provide you with a 30-day meal plan that you can follow. There are lots of tasty recipes that you can try and you can find the recipes for all of them inside this guidebook. Whether you are looking for something light on the run or something that is a bit heartier for at night, you are sure to find many recipes that you can love on this list.

So try a few of them out, or use this as your meal planner, and get ready to find out just how great Weight Watchers can be and just how much weight you can lose.

Day One:	Breakfast: Pancakes = 6 Lunch: Creamy Pesto Pasta = 7 Dinner: Spinach and Chicken Casserole = 4 Total Points: 17 Points
Day Two:	Breakfast: Healthy Morning Cookies = 2 Lunch: BBQ Pork Sandwich = 5 Dinner: Vegetable Quesadilla = 9 Total Points: 16 Points

Day Three:	Breakfast: Cinnamon Rolls = 6 Lunch: Italian Chicken = 5 Dinner: Veggie Pork Chops = 6 Total Points: 17 Points
Day Four:	Breakfast Mushroom and Spinach Quchie = 3 Lunch: Baked Tortellini = 6 Dinner: Cheese Tuna Sandwich = 10 : Total Points: 19 Points
Day Five:	Breakfast: Apple Muffin: 7 Lunch: Cheesy Mushrooms = 2 Dinner: Cheeseburger Soup = 9 : Total Points:17 Points
Day Six	Breakfast: Potato and Cheese Casserole = 7 Lunch: Baked Burrito = 6 Dinner: Beef Chili = 3 : Total Points: 15 Points
Day Seven	Breakfast: Crispy Apple Surprise = 11 Lunch: Veggie Soup = 1 Dinner: Cilantro Lime Shrimp = 3 Total Points: 15 Points
Day Eight:	Breakfast: Breakfast Jelly Pudding = 11 Lunch: Veggie Soup = 1 Dinner: Spinach and Chicken Crescents = 4

	: Total Points:16 Points
Day Nine	Pumpkin Muffins = 4 Lunch: Italian Bread and Tuna Salad = 10 Dinner: Cheesy Chicken Cops = 3 : Total Points:17 Points
Day Ten:	Breakfast: Blackberry and Peach Smoothie = 9 Lunch: Cheeseburger Soup = 7 Dinner Cilantro Lime Shrimp = 3 : Total Points: 19 Points
Day eleven:	Breakfast: Morning Burritos = 9 Lunch: Pasta Veggies = 5 Dinner:Jalapeno Chicken = 4 : Total Points: 18 Points
Day Twelve	Breakfast Souffle = 3 Lunch: Turkey and Cheese Sandwich = 10 Dinner: Jalapeno Chicken = 4 : Total Points: 17 Points
Day thirteen	Breakfast: Breakfast Bars = 6 Lunch: Creamy Pesto Pasta = 7 Dinner: Honey Salmon = 4 : Total Points:17 Points

Day Fourteen	Breakfast: French Toast = 3 Lunch: Baked Fish = 5 Dinner: Mexican Casserole = 8 : Total Points: 16 Points
Day fifteen:	Breakfast: Cheese and Ham Omelet = 6 Lunch: Beef Ziti Bake = 7 Dinner: Cheesy Chicken Chops = 3 : Total Points:16 Points
Day sixteen:	Breakfast: Spiced Honey Cake = 7 Lunch: Chicken Salad = 4 Diner: Veggie Pork Chops = 6 : Total Points: 17 Points
Day seventeen	Breakfast: Blueberry Muffins = 5 Lunch:: BBQ Pork Sandwich = 5 Dinner: Steak and Mashed Potatoes = 9 : Total Points: 18 Pointes
Day eighteen	Breakfast: Yogurt Fluff = 2 Lunch: Baked Fish = 5 Dinner: Pita Bread Pizza =9 : Total Points: 16 Points
Day nineteen	Breakfast: Pancakes = 6 Lunch: Bacon Wraps = 8 Dinner: Egg Salad = 4 : Total Points: 19 Points

Day twenty	Breakfast: Healthy Morning Cookies = 2 Lunch: Beef Burgers = 4 Dinner: Roast Beef with Veggies = 9 : Total Points: 14 Points
Day twenty-one	Breakfast: Cinnamon Rolls = 6 Lunch: Cheesy Mushrooms = 2 Dinner: Cheese and Tuna Sandwich = 10 : Total Points: 18 Points
Day twenty-two	Breakfast: Mushroom and Spinach Quiche = 3 Lunch: Beef Ziti Bake = 7 Dinner: Vegetable Quesadilla = 9 : Total Points 19 Points
Day twenty-three	Breakfast: Apple Muffin = 7 Lunch: Chicken Salad = 4 Dinner: Chicken Thai Wrap =2 : Total Points: 13 Points
Day twenty-four	Breakfast: Potato and Cheese Casserole = 7 Lunch: Bacon wrap = 8 Dinner: Beef Chili = 2 : Total Points: 19 Points
Day twenty-five	Breakfast: Pumpkin Muffins = 4

	Lunch: Italian Bread with Tuna Salad = 10 Dinner: Cola Chicken = 5 Total Points 19 Points
Day twenty-six	Breakfast: Blackberry and Peach Smoothie = 9 Lunch: Beef Burgers = 4 Dinner: Mushroom Steak = 5 : Total Points: 18 Points
Day twenty-seven	Breakfast: Morning Burritos = 9 Lunch: Pasta Veggies = 5 Dinner: Beef Chili = 2 Total Points 18 Points
Day twentyoeght	Breakfast: Breakfast Souffle = 3 Lunch: Baked Burrito = 6 Dinner: Baked Chicken = 10 : Total Points:19 Points
Day twenty-nine	Breakfast: Breakfast Bars = 6 Lunch: Baked Tortellini = 6 Dinner: Potato Soup = 4 Total Points: 18 Points
Day thirty	Breakfast: French Toast = 3 Lunch: Italian Chicken = 5 Dinner: Chicken Dumplings = 9 Total Points = 17 Points

Weight Watchers Breakfasts

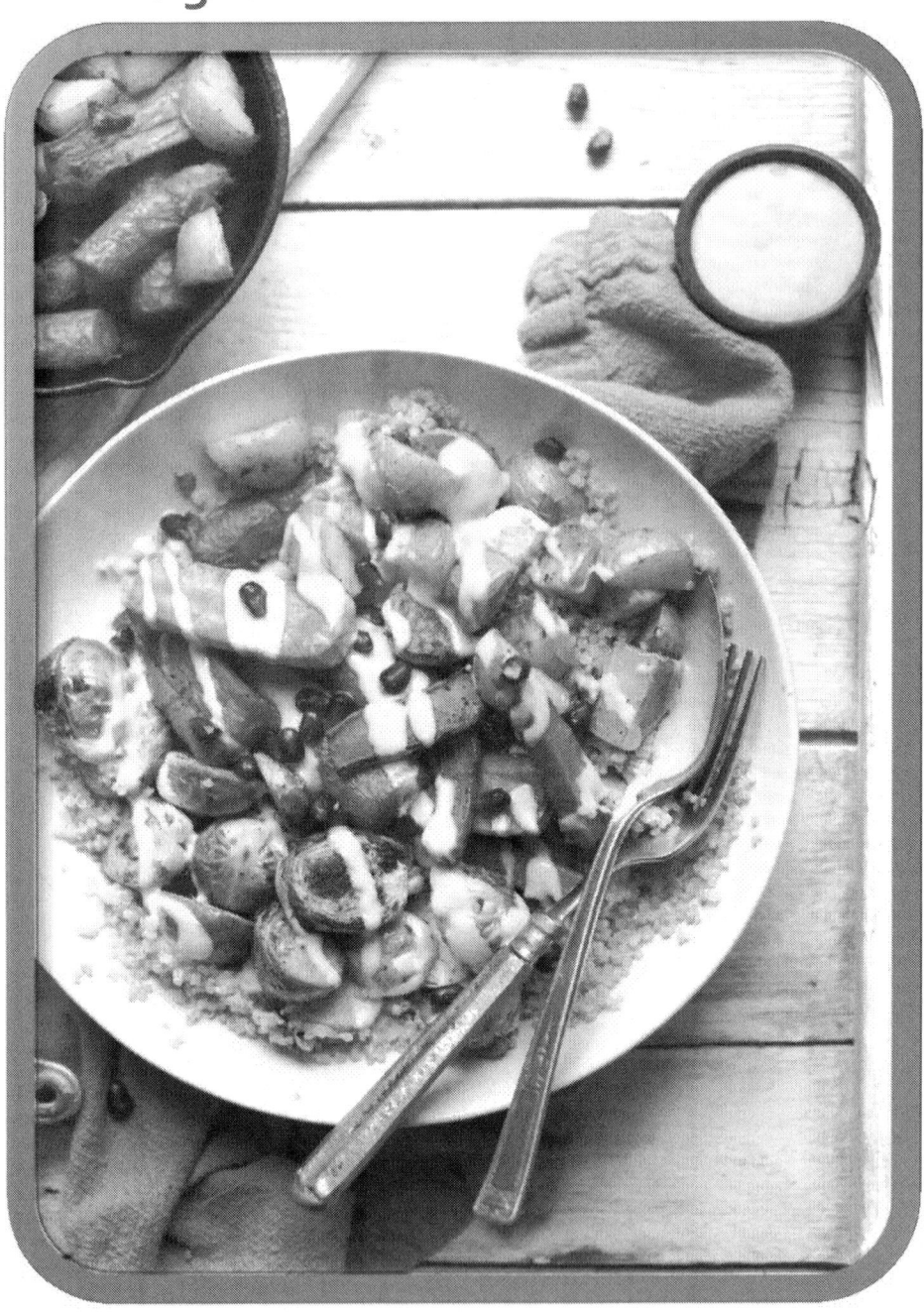

Healthy Pancakes – 6 SmartPoints®

Ingredients:

1 tsp. sweetener, artificial
1 beaten egg white
½ Tbsp. cinnamon
½ Tbsp. baking powder
½ c. buttermilk
¾ c. whole wheat flour
1/3 c. unsweetened applesauce

Directions:

1. Combine together the egg, sweetener, cinnamon, baking powder, buttermilk, flour, and applesauce inside a bowl until there are no more lumps. Add in a bit of water to help the consistency if it is too thick.
2. Spray a bit of cooking spray on the skillet and let it heat up. When the skillet is ready, add a bit of the batter to the skillet and spread it out a bit.
3. Let these pancakes cook for a few minutes to allow the bubbles to start forming.
4. At this time, flip over the pancake and let it cook for an additional minute. Take off the heat when done and then repeat the steps with the rest of the batter until done.

Healthy Morning Cookies – 2 SmartPoints®

Ingredients:

2 egg whites
1/3 c. unsweetened cocoa
1/3 c. chocolate chips, mini
½ c. brown sugar, pressed down
½ c. sugar
1/8 tsp. salt
¼ c. butter, softened
1 c. flour
¼ tsp. baking soda

Directions:

1. Turn on the oven and let it heat up to 350 degrees. Take out a cookie sheet and spray it with some cooking spray.
2. Now take out a bowl and mix together the baking soda, flour, and salt. In a second bowl, combine the butter and the brown sugar and mix together until fluffy.
3. Add in the sugar to this second bowl and continue to beat to make it well incorporated. Put all of this into the flour mixture and keep on stirring to combine. Now add in the chocolate chips.

4. Place small amounts of this onto the cookie sheet and then put into the oven and let it bake for about 10 minutes.
5. Take out of the oven and allow the cookies to cool down for a few minutes before taking them off the pan and cooling down completely.

Cinnamon Rolls—6 SmortPoints

Ingredients:

¼ c. cream cheese
¼ c. sugar
¼ tsp. vanilla
1 tsp. butter, melted
11 oz. breadstick dough, cold
2 Tbsp. brown sugar
1 tsp. cinnamon

Directions:

1. Turn on the oven and let it heat up to 375 degrees. While that is heating up, take out a baking pan and prepare it with some cooking spray.
2. Take out a small bowl and mix together the brown sugar, cinnamon, and the butter and place to the side.
3. Take the breadstick dough and make it into 12 strips. Sprinkle on some brown sugar to this dough and then roll them into a spiral. Press the dough down to seal up the ends.

4. Place these rolls into a baking pan, leaving them about an inch apart. Place into the oven and let them bake for 15 minutes. When they are done, take out of the oven and let them cool for 10 minutes.
5. While the rolls are baking, work on the frosting. Bring out a bowl and mix together the cream cheese, sugar, and vanilla. Add a bit of water to this until you get the consistency that you would like.
6. Drizzle this frosting onto the prepared rolls and let it set for a few minutes before serving.

Mushroom and Spinach Quiche – 3 SmartPoints®

Ingredients:

Salt
Pepper
¼ c. chopped onion
3 eggs
½ c. cottage cheese
2 tsp. garlic, minced
1 c. artichoke hearts, chopped
½ tsp. olive oil
10 oz. spinach
1 c. mushrooms, sliced

Directions:

1. Turn on the oven and let it heat up to 350 degrees. While that is heating up, take out a pan and cook together the olive oil, mushrooms, onions, and garlic.
2. When those are ready, add in the spinach and let it cook for a bit. After a few minutes, add in the rest of the ingredients and season with some pepper and salt.
3. Place this into a prepared pie dish and let it bake for 45 minutes before serving.

Apple Muffin – 7 SmartPoints®

Ingredients:

½ c. milk
2 Tbsp. vegetable oil
½ tsp. salt
½ tsp. cinnamon
1 ½ tsp. baking powder
1 c. oats
½ tsp. baking soda
2/3 c. brown sugar
2 c. shredded apple
1 ½ c. flour, all purpose

Directions:

1. Turn on the oven and let it heat up to 375 degrees. In the meantime, take out a muffin pan and grease it up.

2. Take out a bowl and combine together the milk, cinnamon, vegetable oil, baking soda, salt, brown sugar, baking powder, flour, and oats.
3. When this is all combined, pour the batter inside the muffin tin and then place into the oven.
4. Allow these to bake for 18 minutes or until they are all done. Give them some time to cool down before serving.

Potato and Cheese Casserole – 7 SmartPoints®

Ingredients:

Salt
Pepper
4 beaten eggs
1 can milk, evaporated
3 oz. bacon, chopped
½ c. scallion, sliced
3 c. potato, shredded
¾ c. cheddar cheese

Directions:

1. For this recipe, turn on the oven and let it heat up to 350 degrees. Take out your baking pan and coat it with some cooking spray.
2. Place the potatoes into the prepared baking pan and then top with some cheese, scallions, and bacon.

3. Now bring out a small bowl and mix together the pepper, salt, eggs, and milk inside. Pour this all on top of the potato mixture.
4. Place this meal inside the oven and let it cook for 40 minutes or until everything has time to set.
5. Take it out of the oven and give it a few minutes to cool down before slicing and enjoying.

Crispy Apple Surprise – 11 SmartPoints®

Ingredients:

Ground cloves
3 lb. sliced apples
¼ c. sugar
1 tsp. vanilla
¼ tsp. nutmeg
3 Tbsp. butter
1 tsp. water
¼ tsp. cinnamon
Salt
¼ c. brown sugar
½ tsp. ginger
½ c. and 2 Tbsp. flour
½ c. quick cooking oats

Directions;

1. For this recipe, turn on the oven and let it heat up to 375 degrees. Take out a baking dish and cover it with some cooking spray.

2. First we will need to make the topping. To do this, bring out a bowl and combine the oats with the cinnamon, salt, brown sugar, ginger, and ½ cup of flour.
3. Add in the butter at this time and then place it all into the pastry blender so that you get a nice crumbly mixture. Pour in some water and then press this to make clumps.
4. Now you will want to work on the filling. To do this, bring out a bowl and combine the cloves, sugar, nutmeg, and the rest of the flour. Put in the vanilla and the apples in as well and then pour everything inside a baking dish.
5. Pour your topping over the filling and then place everything into the oven. Bake this all in the oven for 60 minutes.

Breakfast Jelly Pudding – 11 SmartPoints®
Ingredients:

16 oz. fruit cocktail, canned
16 oz. mandarin orange, canned
1/3 oz. raspberry Jell-O, sugar free
20 oz. pineapple, canned
16 oz. whipped cream
1 oz. vanilla pudding mix

Directions:

1. Take out the canned fruits and take all of the liquid out of them. Bring out a bowl and

combine the pudding mix, gelatin, and whipped cream.
2. Slowly fold in the fruits that you just drained out and then chill for a few hours inside the fridge before serving.

Pumpkin Muffins – 4 SmartPoints®

Ingredients:

18 oz. spice cake mix
15 oz. pumpkin
1 c. water

Directions:

1. For this recipe, turn on the oven and let it heat up to 375 degrees.
2. While the oven is heating up, take out a bowl and combine the water, pumpkin, and spice cake mix.
3. Prepare a muffin pan and then pour the batter inside of it. Place these into the oven and bake until it is all done before serving.

Blackberry and Peach Smoothie – 9 SmartPoints®

Ingredients:

½ c. skim milk
¾ c. ice cubes
¼ c. blackberries
2 peeled peaches, sliced

Directions:

1. Bring out a blender and add in the milk, ice cubes, blackberries, and peaches.
2. Turn on the blender and let it process all of the ingredients until they are smooth.
3. Pour this into your favorite cup and then serve!

Morning Burritos – 9 SmartPoints®

Ingredients:

½ c. sour cream
½ c. salsa
¼ tsp. pepper
4 tortillas
2 Tbsp. cilantro
¼ tsp. salt
4 egg whites
½ c. cheddar cheese
2 chopped garlic cloves
2 eggs

1 diced green pepper
½ c. tomato, chopped
2 tsp. olive oil
1/3 c. scallions, chopped

Directions:

1. To start this recipe, turn on the oven and let it heat up to 400 degrees. Take out a baking pan and spray it with some cooking spray.
2. Now you can add in a bit of oil to the skillet and add in the tomato garlic, scallions, and green pepper. Let this cook for about 5 minutes.
3. After this time, add in the eggs and the egg whites and cook for another five minutes. Take everything off the heat at this time.
4. Add in the salt, pepper, cheese, and cilantro.
5. Lay out the tortillas and scoop a bit of the filling into each one. Roll them up tight and then place into the baking pan.
6. Bake these in the oven for 10 minutes. Serve with a bit of salsa and some sour cream and then enjoy!

Breakfast Souffle – 3 SmartPoints®

Ingredients:

1/8 tsp. cayenne pepper

2 eggs

2 egg whites

1 ½ c. cheddar cheese

½ tsp. salt

3 Tbsp. flour

1 c. milk

Directions:

1. Take out a bowl and mix three tablespoons of the milk together with the flour and set to the side.
2. Place the rest of the milk into a pan and let it cook over a low heat. Add the flour mixture to this pan and then cook it while stirring the whole time so that it can begin to thicken.
3. Remove this from the heat and then put in a bit of salt and the cayenne pepper and cheese. Move this over to a bowl and let it cool down.
4. Turn on the oven on to 350 degrees. While that is heating up, add the egg yolks into the cheese mixture until they are well incorporated.
5. Bring out a glass bowl and whip up all the egg whites together. Combine ¼ of these with the cheese mixture and then fold in the rest of the beaten egg with our rubber spatula.
6. Place this mixture into a soufflé dish and then bake in the oven for about 35 minutes. Serve right away when it is done.

Breakfast Bars – 6 SmartPoints®

Ingredients:

1 tsp. vailla
1/3 c. water
¾ c. chocolate chips
6 Tbsp. butter
2 egg whites
½ tsp. salt
2 c. flour
2 tsp. baking powder

Directions:

1. Turn on the oven and let it heat up to 350 degrees. While that is heating up, bring out a bowl and mix together the salt, baking powder, and flour.
2. In another bowl, mix together the butter and the brown sugar until the are nice and fluffy before adding in the egg whites and the vanilla. Slowly whisk in the flour mixture and alternate it with a bit of water as well.
3. Add in the chocolate chips and mix them in well. Place some foil onto a baking pan and then pour the mixture on the pan.
4. Place this into the oven and let it bake for 25 minutes. Let the bars cool on a wire wrack when you are done. Cut into slices when you are ready and enjoy.

Tasty French Toast – 3 SmartPoints®

Ingredients:

6 slices wheat bread
1 pkg. sugar free maple syrup
1 Tbsp. cinnamon
1 Tbsp. vanilla
Cooking spray
4 egg whites
¼ c. skim milk

Directions:

1. To start this recipe, bring out a bowl and mix together the egg whites and the vanilla.
2. Take out a skillet and grease it u with some cooking spray. Heat up the skillet.
3. While the skillet is heating up, dip the bread slices in the egg mixture and let each side get nice and soaked. Allow the extra batter to drip off.
4. Place the bread onto the skillet and let each side cook for about 3 minutes. Place these onto a plate and serve.

Cheese and Ham Omelet – 6 SmartPoints®

Ingredients:

½ c. diced ham
¼ c. Parmesan cheese

1/8 tsp. pepper
1/8 tsp. hot pepper sauce
2 Tbsp. green onion, chopped
¼ tsp. salt
2 eggs
4 egg whites

Directions:

1. For this recipe, bring out a bowl and ix together the hot sauce, salt, pepper, eggs, and onion.
2. Take out a skillet and grease it with some cooking spray before heating it up. Pour the mixture into the skillet and let it cook for 5 minutes so it has time to set.
3. Sprinkle the top with the ham and the Parmesan cheese. Fold the omelet in half and let it cook for another minute before serving.

Spiced Honey Cake – 7 SmartPoints®

Ingredients:

1 tsp. grated orange zest
2 Tbsp. canola oil
½ c. honey
¼ c. sliced almonds
2 eggs
¼ c. white sugar
½ tsp. nutmeg
½ tsp. cloves
1 tsp. cinnamon

¾ tsp. allspice
½ tsp. baking soda
1/8 tsp. salt
1 ½ c. flour
¾ tsp. baking powder
½ c. applesauce

Directions:

1. To start this recipe, turn on the oven and let it heat up to 350 degrees. Grease up a loaf pan using some cooking spray and set it to the side.
2. Mix together the nutmeg, cloves, cinnamon, allspice, baking soda, salt, four, and baking powder. When this is combined, set it aside.
3. In another bowl, beat together the eggs until the are frothy. Add in the sugar, honey, and oil and mix to make this a pale yellow before adding in the orange zest and apple sauce.
4. Slowly combined in the wet mixture and the dry mixture, making sure to combine them together well. When these are read, pour inside a loaf pan and then top with some almonds.
5. Place all of this into the oven and let it bake for about 40 minutes until it is cooked all the way through.
6. Allow the cake to cool down for another 20 minutes before serving.

Blueberry Muffins – 5 SmartPoints®

Ingredients:

2 ½ c. hot water
1 ½ tsp. baking powder
3 c. bran cereal
19 oz. blueberry muffin mix

Directions:

1. Turn on the oven and let it heat up to 400 degrees. Prepare a muffin pan using some paper liners or with some cooking spray.
2. While the oven is heating up, combine the hot water and the bran cereal together and then set them to the side.
3. Bring out another bowl so that you can mix together the baking powder and the muffin mix. When these are combined, place the bran cereal and water so that they can be incorporated as well.
4. Pour this batter inside of your prepared muffin pan and then bake for 15 minutes or until the muffins are cooked all the way through.

Yogurt Fluff – 2 SmartPoints®

Ingredients:

12 tsp. vanilla
Ice cubes
½ c. cold water
1 c. yogurt
¾ c. boiling water
8 ½ grams cherry gelatin

Directions:

1. Combine together the gelatin and the boiling water inside of a bowl and ix so that the gelatin is completely dissolved.
2. Put the ice cubes into some cold water and then get a cup of this mixture. Pour this into the gelatin and continue to mix so that it can become thicker. Get rid of any ice that is extra.
3. Add in the yogurt as well as the vanilla and let it stir until it becomes well blended.
4. Place the bowl into the fridge and let it chill for at least 30 minutes. After this time add in some whipped cream and enjoy!

Weight Watchers Lunches

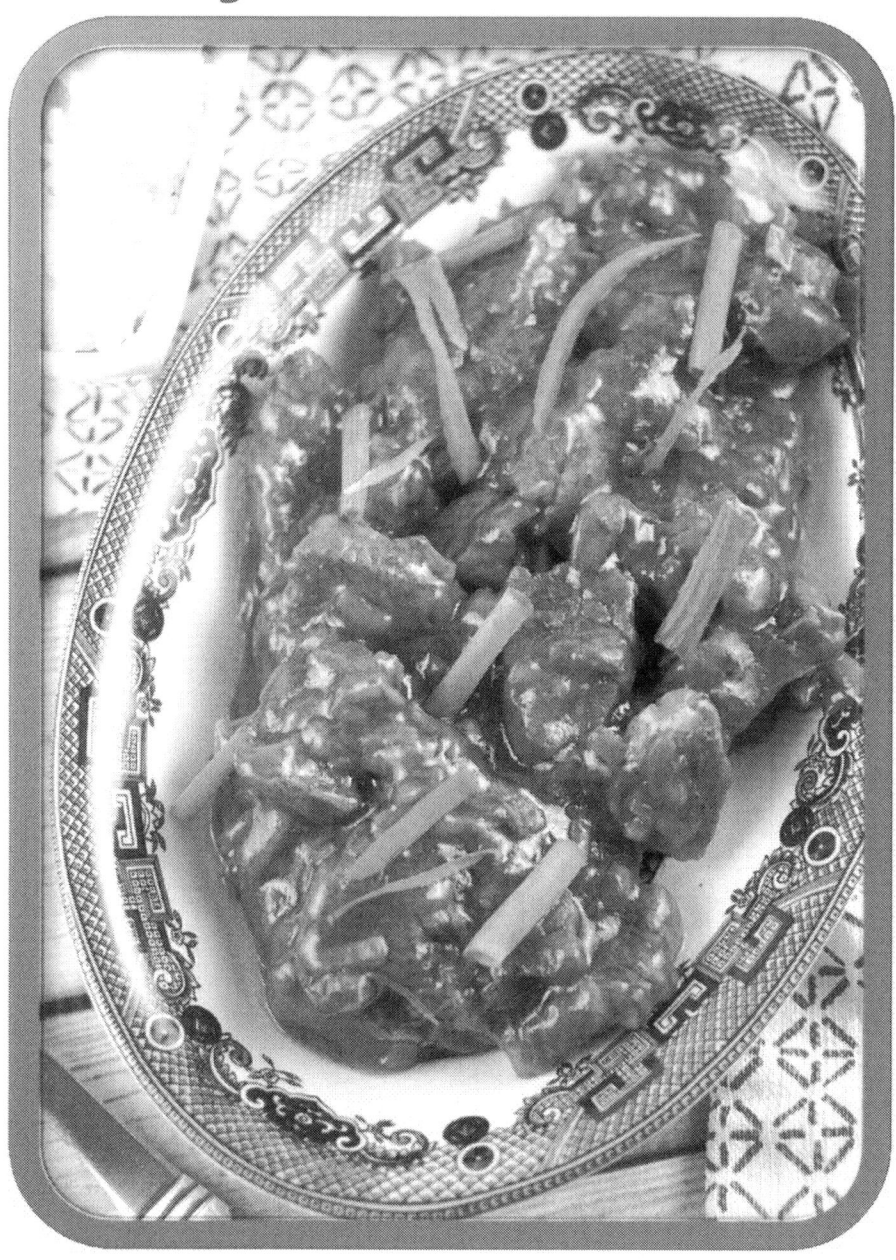

Creamy Pesto Pasta – 7 SmartPoints®

Ingredients:

1 tsp. lemon juice
1 ½ tsp. olive oil
2 ½ Tbsp. cream cheese
2 garlic cloves
4 ½ c. baby spinach
2 Tbsp. water
1 ¼ tsp. salt
8 oz. uncooked spaghetti

Directions:

1. For this recipe, take out a pot of water and boil it with a bit of salt. Add in the pasta and let it cook for 8 minutes or until it is all done.
2. Drain out the water and top with some cherry tomatoes and Parmesan cheese. Process the salt, oil, garlic, spinach, and water inside the blender until it is soft.
3. Add in the cream cheese to the pasta until it melts. Then add in the reserved pasta water and the pesto sauce and mix to get the right consistency.
4. Season with some lemon juice and salt and then enjoy.

BBQ Pork Sandwich – 5 SmartPoints®

Ingredients:
1 cut bell pepper, green
6 hamburger buns
12 oz. pork tenderloin
¼ tsp. salt
1 tsp. Worcestershire sauce
1 Tbsp. brown sugar
1 ½ tsp. chili powder
6 oz. can tomato paste
2 Tbsp. red wine vinegar
2 minced garlic cloves
2/3 c. water
1 minced onion

Directions:
1. Grease up a small pan with some cooking spray and then heat it up. Add in the onion and the garlic and let these cook for 5 minutes.
2. At this time, add in the oregano, Worcestershire sauce, brown sugar, chili powder, tomato paste, vinegar, and garlic. Bring all of this to a boil.
3. Simmer this without the top on for about 10 minutes so that the liquid can reduce a bt, making sure to stir occasionally.
4. While that is cooking, take the meat and remove the fat a bit. Cut this meat into smaller strips. Take out another skillet and brush with some cooking spray.
5. Season the meat with some salt and place the meat in the skillet. Cook the meat for three

minutes before pouring in the bell peppers and sauce.
6. Cook all of the ingredients together for a few minutes. When it is ready, serve the pork on toasted buns and enjoy.

Italian Chicken – 5 SmartPoints®

Ingredients:
Juice from two lemons
Pepper
Salt
2 Tbsp. capers
¼ c. parsley, chopped
½ c. chicken broth
2 Tbsp. butter
1 ½ lbs. chicken breast, sliced
¾ c. white wine

Directions:
1. To start up this recipe, turn on the oven and let it heat up to 350 degrees. Lay out the chicken breasts onto a board and then cover with some cling wrap. Flatten the chicken with a mallet to make them ¼ inch thick.
2. Season the chicken with the pepper and salt and then move this over to a baking dish. Add some butter to the chicken and then surround it with the broth, wine, and lemon juice.
3. Sprinkle everything with the capers and then cover with some foil before placing into the oven and baking for 20 minutes.

4. Remove the foil after this time and then bake them for an additional 10 minutes. Sprinkle with some parsley and then serve right away.

Baked Tortellini – 6 SmartPoints®

Ingredients:

2/3 c. mozzarella cheese
2 tsp. lemon zest
2 c. spinach
¼ tsp. red pepper flakes
1 Tbsp. lemon juice
1/8 tsp. pepper
1 ½ tsp. basil
¾ tsp. salt
2 Tbsp. flour
2 c. milk
2 bacon slices
3 chopped garlic cloves
12 oz. dry spinach and cheese
1 pkg. tortellini
1 ½ oz. Parmesan cheese

Directions:

1. Turn on the oven and let it heat up to 350 degrees. While that is heating up, take out a baking dish and cover with some cooking spray.
2. Follow the directions on the package and cook the tortellini. In the meantime, place the bacon into a skillet and cook for 9 minutes so it

becomes crisp. Take the bacon off the skillet and put on a paper towel to absorb the oil. Save some of this bacon grease.
3. Add the garlic into the bacon grease and let it cook for a minute before adding in the flour and whisk in the milk. Now add in the basil, red pepper flakes, and pepper.
4. Bring all of this to a simmer and then add in the lemon juice and lemon zest and let t stir for another 3 minutes.
5. Take all of this off the heat. Crumble up the bacon and set it to the side. Mix the mozzarella, spinach, parmesan, and tortellini together.
6. Move this mixture to the baking dish and top with the rest of the bacon, Parmesan, and mozzarella.
7. Cover this with foil and place into the oven to bake for 20 minutes. Remove the foil at this time and then bake for another 10 minutes before serving.

Cheesy Mushrooms – 2 SmartPoints®

Ingredients:

½ tsp. olive oil
1/8 tsp. cayenne pepper
1 tsp. lemon juice
½ tsp. lemon zest
2 Tbsp. feta cheese
½ Tbsp. parsley
8 mushrooms
2 pieces mushroom stems

Directions:

1. Turn on the oven and let it heat up to 425 degrees. Bring out a baking dish and let it get covered with cooking spray.
2. Rinse the mushrooms and dry them with some paper towels. Pull the stems off the mushrooms and set two of these to the side. Mince up the mushroom stems and place into a bowl.
3. Place the mushrooms into the baking dish and then mx in the rest of the ingredients with the minced stems. Place this mixture into the caps of the mushrooms.
4. Place this into the oven and let it bake for about 15 minutes. Allow this some time to cool down before serving.

Baked Burrito – 6 SmartPoints®

Ingredients:

¼ c. water
1 c. Mexican cheese
10 oz. canned refried beans
1 c. Bisquick
1 c. mozzarella cheese
1 lb. ground beef
1 pack taco seasoning

Directions:

1. Cook up the ground beef and until it is cooked all the way through and then drain out the liquid. Add in the taco seasoning and let it simmer.
2. Bring out another bowl and combine the refried beans with the Bisquick and water. Put this mixture into a pan and then top with some cheese and beef.
3. Turn on the oven to 350 degrees and then add in the meal. Bake this for 30 minutes and then serve.

Italian Bread with some Tuna Salad – 10 SmartPoints®

Ingredients:

8 oz. Italian bread
2 tomatoes, sliced
¼ tsp. salt
1 tsp. dried oregano
½ tsp. pepper
3 Tbsp. balsamic vinegar
1 red onion, sliced
1 Tbsp. capers, rinsed or drained.
4 c. lettuce, shredded
8 oz. white tuna

Directions:

1. Start by making the tuna salad part. Mix together the onion, capers, lettuce, and tuna. Set this to the side.
2. Then you can go on and make the dressing. To do this, you will be able to mix together the salt, pepper, garlic, oregano, vinegar, olive oil. Drizzle this on top of the tuna salad and toss around to combine.
3. Next it is time to make the sandwiches. You can cut the bread lengthwise and then spread it open. Arrange the tomatoes on the bottom of the bread.
4. Top this all with the salad mixture and then wrap up the sandwich with some cling wrap. Chill in the fridge for a few hours before serving.

Turkey and Cheese Sandwich – 10 SmartPoints®

Ingredients:

8 slices of bread
4 oz. sliced cheese
½ c. milk
4 tsp. Dijon mustard
4 oz. sliced chicken breast
1 egg
1 egg white

Directions:

1. Take out a small bowl and whisk together the milk, egg, and egg white. Lay out the bread and layer with some of the mustard on top.
2. Top the bread slices with some turkey and cheese. Put the rest of the bread slices on top of them to put the sandwiches together.
3. Grease a pan with some cooking spray and then place over the heat. Coat each of the sandwiches with the egg mixture and place inside a hot pan.
4. Cook the sandwiches for about 4 minutes on each side before serving.

Delicious Veggie Soup – 1 SmartPoint

Ingredients:

1 tsp. Cajun spices
¼ tsp. basil
2 beef bouillon cubs
½ c. zucchini slices
2 minced garlic cloves
14 ½ oz. canned tomatoes, diced
2 ½ c. cabbage, shredded
1 ½ stalks chopped celery
14 oz. canned beef broth
½ sliced onion
1 c. sliced carrot

Directions:

1. Spray a pan with some cooking spray and then add inn the celery, onions, and carrots inside.
2. Take out a big pot and mx together the basil, garlic, Cajun spice, cabbage, bouillon cubes, beef broth, and tomatoes together. Add in the vegetables you just cooked as well.
3. Bring all of this to a boil and let it simmer together for about 30 minutes.
4. After this time, put the zucchini into the pot and simmer for an additional 10 minutes. Serve it warm.

Cheeseburger Soup – 7 SmartPoints®

Ingredients:

1/8 tsp. pepper
24 pieces corn tortilla chips
½ tsp. paprika
¼ tsp. salt
1 c. evaporated milk
8 oz. cubed Velveeta
2 Tbsp. flour
3 c. chicken broth
1 chopped celery stalk
1 lb. uncooked ground beef
1 chopped garlic clove
1 diced onion
Cooking spray

Directions:

1. Take out a skillet and spray on some cooking spray. Add on the celery, garlic, and onion and let these cook until they are tender.
2. Bring out a slow cooker and spray with some cooking spray. Transfer these over to the slow cooker.
3. Take out another skillet and cook the beef for about six minutes or until it is cooked through. Move this over to the slow cooker.
4. In another bowl, mix together ½ cup of the broth so that you can get rid of the lumps. Put

the flour into the skillet and add in the rest 2 ½ cups of broth inside.
5. Let this simmer, taking time to take the browned bits off the bottom of the skillet. When this is done, move it over to the slow cooker and add in the pepper, paprika, salt, evaporated milk, and cheese.
6. Place the lid into the slow cooker and let it cook on a low setting for 2 hours. Pour your flour mixture inside the slow cooker at this time.
7. Cover the slow cooker and let this cook for another 15 minutes. When you are ready to serve, add some crushed tortilla chips and enjoy.

Pasta Veggies – 5 SmartPoints®

Ingredients:

½ c. mayo
2 Tbsp. scallions, sliced
½ tsp. red pepper
¼ c. celery, diced
¾ c. salsa
½ yellow bell pepper
½ c. cherry tomatoes
6 oz. pasta
12 oz. tuna, canned

Directions:

1. Cook the pasta by following the directions on the package. When this is done, drain out the pasta and rinse it under some cold water. Then drain it again.
2. Now you can bring out a big bowl and mix together the celery, bell pepper, tomatoes, pasta, and tuna.
3. In a second bowl, combine the red pepper, salsa, and mayo together. Pour this dressing over the pasta mixture and toss it together well.
4. Cover the bowl and then place into the fridge to chill for a bit. Right before serving, top with some scallions and enjoy.

Bacon Wrap – 8 SmartPoints®

Ingredients:

½ lb. sliced roast beef
2 sliced tomatoes
¼ tsp. pepper
7 pieces tortilla
2 tsp. Dijon mustard
2 c. shredded lettuce
¼ tsp. salt
1/3 c. basil
1/3 c. mayo

Directions:

1. Bring out a bowl and combine the pepper, Dijon mustard, salt, basil, and mayo.
2. Lay out the tortillas and spread the mixture from above all over it.
3. Sprinkle the tortillas with some lettuce, roast beef, and tomatoes. Roll this up and then serve.

Cornmeal Baked Fish – 5 SmartPoints®

Ingredients:

½ tsp. paprika
1/3 c. milk
½ tsp. salt
3 Tbsp. melted butter
1/8 tsp. pepper
¼ c. bread crumbs
½ tsp. dill
1 ½ lb. white fish fillet
¼ c. yellow cornmeal

Directions:

1. Turn on the oven and let it heat up to 450 degrees. Bring out a pie plate and combine together all of your dry ingredients.
2. Add in the milk to another milk. Dip the fish inside the milk to coat and then put it through the crumb mixture.
3. Place the fish into a greased pan and then drizzle the fish with some melted butter.

4. Bake the fish for 10 minutes and then serve with your favorite sides.

Beef Ziti Bake – 7 SmartPoints®

Ingredients:

20 oz. crushed tomatoes
1 c. mozzarella cheese
1 tsp. oregano
1 tsp. thyme
¼ tsp. pepper
1/3 lb. ground beef
½ tsp. salt
2 minced garlic cloves
12 oz. ziti
2 tsp. olive oil

Directions:

1. Turn on the oven and let it heat up to 350 degrees. Cook the ziti by following the directions on the package. When this is done, drain out the pasta and rinse it off.
2. Heat up some olive oil into a pan and then cook the garlic inside for a minute. Cook the ground beef in here, seasoning with some pepper and salt, and cook all the way through.
3. Remove the fat and then mix in the thyme, rosemary, and oregano and cook for two more

minutes. Add in the tomatoes and bring to a boil to simmer for five minutes.
4. Bring out a casserole dish and put some of the meat sauce to cover all of the bottom. Put in half of your prepared ziti and then the rest of the meat sauce. Now add in half of the mozzarella cheese and then finish the layers.
5. Bake the ziti in the oven for 30 minutes so the cheese has time to melt the cheese before serving.

Chicken Salad – 4 SmartPoints®

Ingredients:

½ tsp. salt
¼ tsp. pepper
1 tsp. Dijon mustard
1 tsp. lemon juice
2 Tbsp. sour cream
2 Tbsp. parsley
1/3 c. dill pickle
¼ c. mayo
1 lb. chicken breast
½ c. celery, chopped

Directions:

1. Take out a pan and place the chicken inside. Add in just enough water to cover up the chicken. Bring this all to a boil.

2. Allow the chicken to boil for 10 minutes and then drain out the liquid, allowing the chicken to cool a bit.
3. Slice the chicken into small cubes and then place the chicken into a bowl.
4. At this time, add in the pepper, salt, lemon juice, parsley, mustard, mayo, sour cream, celery, and pickles together. Toss around to coat and serve.

Egg Salad – 4 SmartPoints®

Ingredients:

¼ tsp. pepper
½ tsp. salt
1 piece of dill
2 Tbsp. mayo
½ tsp. Dijon mustard
2 Tbsp. chives
4 eggs
2 hard boiled eggs

Directions:

1. Bring out a pan and fill it with the water and the eggs. Place this on a high heat and bring it to a boil.
2. When the eggs are done, drain the water out and add in the eggs to an ice water bath. When the eggs are cooled down, you can remove the shells from the eggs.

3. Also take some time to remove the yolks from two the eggs. Slice up the eggs into smaller pieces and add into a bowl.
4. Add in the pepper, salt, mustard, dill, chives, and mayo to the bowl and stir well before serving.

Beef Burgers – 4 SmartPoints®

Ingredients;

½ tsp. salt
¼ tsp. pepper
Four hamburger buns, low calorie
1 Tbsp. Worcestershire sauce
2 tsp. garlic, minced
Cooking spray
1 lb. ground beef

Directions:

1. Coat your griddle with some cooking spray and heat it up. Take out a bowl and add in the pepper, salt, Worcestershire sauce, garlic, and beef. Form this into patties.
2. Place the burgers onto the prepared griddle and cook the patties for five minutes on each side.
3. Add some of our favorite toppings and then enjoy.

Dinners on Weight Watchers For The Whole Family

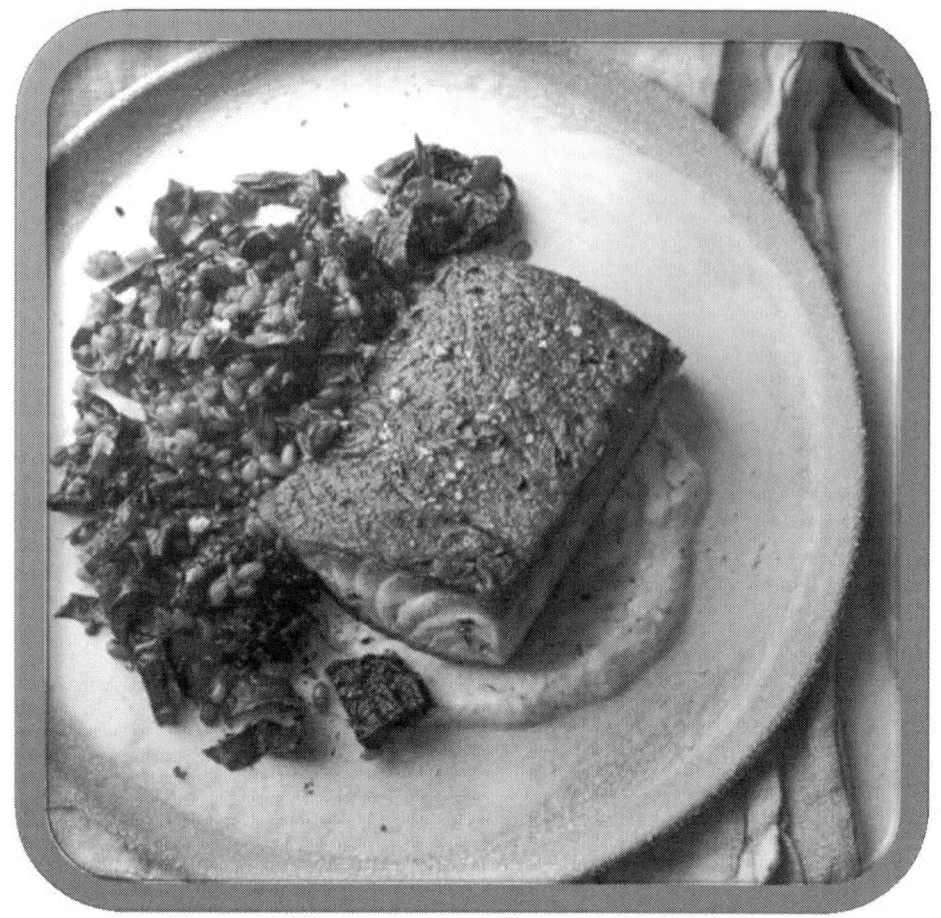

Cheesy Chicken Chops == 3 Smart Points
Ingredients:

½ tsp. garlic powder
¼ tsp. pepper
1 lb. chicken breast

1/8 tsp. paprika
1 tsp. parsley
¼ c. parmesan cheese
2 Tbsp. dried Italian bread crumbs

Directions:

1. Turn on the oven and let it heat up to 400 degrees. Bring out a bag and add in the seasonings, cheese, and crumbs and mix them together.
2. Move this mixture over to a plate. Coat the chicken in this cheese mixture and then move over to a baking sheet.
3. Allow this to bake inside the air fryer for about 25 minutes or until it is cooked through and then serve.

Jalapeno Chicken – 5 SmartPoints®

Ingredients:

2 Tbsp. Worcestershire sauce
16 oz. chicken breasts
1 tsp. garlic powder
1/3 c. steak sauce
1/3 c. jalapeno jelly, melted

Directions:

1. Bring out a small bowl and mix together the Worcestershire sauce, garlic powder, steak sauce, and jalapeno jelly.

2.   Add the chicken into this mixture and let it marinate inside the fridge overnight.

3.   Spray the griddle with some cooking spray. Cook the chicken for about 5 minutes on each side so that the chicken can cook through.

Cilantro Lime Shrimp – 3 SmartPoints®

Ingredients:

¼ tsp. pepper
¼ c. cilantro, chopped
1 tsp. lime zest, grated
2 minced garlic cloves
1 Tbsp. olive oil
½ tsp. cumin
¼ tsp. ginger
1 ¾ lb. shrimp
2 Tbsp. lime juice
½ tsp. salt

Directions;

1.   To make this simple recipe, bring out a bowl and mix together the garlic, cumin, ginger, shrimp, and lime juice.

2.   Heat up some oil inside a skillet and then add in the shrimp. Let it cook inside the skillet for about 4 minutes.

3.   Before serving, garnish with some pepper, salt, cilantro, and lime zest.

Spinach and Chicken Crescents == 4 SmartPoints®

Ingredients:

1 c. baby spinach
1/3 c. Mexican blend cheese
5 oz. chicken strips, grilled
8 oz. crescent roll dough
4 Tbsp. cream cheese, soft

Directions:

1. Turn on the oven and let it heat up to 375 degrees. Put the crescent rolls onto a baking sheet and put some spinach and cream cheese on top of the rolls.
2. Grill up the chicken strips if you need to and then place these on the crescent with the Mexican cheese.
3. Tuck in the roll to wrap up the filling and then bake the meal for about 14 minutes inside the oven before serving.

Steak and Mashed Potatoes – 8 SmartPoints®

Ingredients;

1 ½ c. beef broth
4 cube steaks
Pepper
8 oz. sliced mushrooms
4 Tbsp. flour

1 lb. diced potatoes
½ tsp. salt

Directions:

1. To start this recipe, bring out a pot and boil and simmer the potatoes until they are nice and tender. Drain these out when you are done and keep ½ cup of the liquid.
2. Season the cooked potatoes with some pepper and salt and then mash them up using the liquid that you reserved.
3. Mix together some of the extra liquid with 2 tablespoon flour. Cover the steaks with the remaining flour as well as some salt and pepper and then cook the steaks for about 2 minutes on each side.
4. Mix in the mushrooms to this mixture and bring it all to a boil. When it reaches a boil, simmer the ingredients for 30 minutes.
5. Remove the cover at this time and cook so the gravy can thicken. Serve with some of the mashed potatoes and enjoy.

Honey Salmon – 4 SmartPoints®

Ingredients:

½ tsp. pepper
¼ c. sliced scallions
1 lb. salmon fillets
½ tsp. salt
1 tsp. ginger

2 tsp. wasabi
1 Tbsp. soy sauce
1 Tbsp. honey
3 Tbsp. mirin
1 Tbsp. rice vinegar

Direction:

1. Boil the wasabi, ginger, soy sauce, honey, mirin, and vinegar together in a pan for about five minutes.
2. After this time, take it off the heat and sprinkle with some salt and pepper. Sprinkle with a bit of salt and pepper.
3. Grease up a skillet and let it heat up a little bit. Cook the salmon in the skillet on 4 minutes on both sides.
4. Spoon a bit of the sauce on top of the salmon and then top a bit of the scallions on top of it before serving.

Veggie Pork Chops – 6 SmartPoints®

Ingredients:

1 ½ tsp. oregano
½ tsp. cumin
2 c. corn
½ c. salsa
1 diced onion
14.5 oz. can stewed tomatoes
16 oz. pork chops
1 diced green peppers

Directions:

1. Turn the oven on and let it heat up to 350 degrees. Cook up the pork chops in a preheated skillet and let it cook for two minutes on each side of the meat.
2. Move the pork over to a prepared casserole dish. Grease up the skillet with some more cooking spray and then add in the rest of the ingredients. Cook these for about five minutes.
3. When these ingredients are well combined, pour this mixture all over the pork chops and then cover the dish with some foil.
4. Bake the pork chops in the oven for about 50 minutes or until the pork is cooked through before serving.

Mexican Casserole – 8 SmartPoints®

Ingredients:

1/3 c. Mexican cheese blend
1/3 chopped cilantro bunch
8 pieces corn tortilla
¾ c. sour cream
15 oz. corn kernels
15 oz. can black beans
¼ c. jalapeno pepper, chopped
2 c. tomato, chopped
1 lb. ground beef
½ c. diced onion

Directions:

1. Bring out our skillet and cook the onions and beef inside for about 12 minutes. Drain and rinse off the meat with some warm water in order to remove some of the fat.
2. Place the meat into the skillet again and add in the taco seasoning mix, tomatoes, jalapenos, corn, and black beans and let this heat and simmer for another five minutes.
3. Cut the 8 tortillas in half and then arrange 8 of the halves into a prepared baking dish. Put half of the beef mixture and the sour cream over the tortillas.
4. Cover with the rest of the tortillas and then the rest of the beef mixture. Turn the oven on to 350 degrees at this time.
5. Bake the dish for about 25 minutes. When this is all done, top with some cilantro and cheese before serving.

Chicken Thai Wrap – 2 SmartPoints®

Ingredients:

½ tsp. grated ginger
1 handful sliced green onions
½ tsp. soy sauce
Hot sauce
1/3 c. cabbage
¼ c. snap peas

1/3 c. red bell pepper strips
2 Tbsp. PB2
1 wheat wrap
2 oz. chicken breast

Directions:

1. Start this recipe by bringing out a bowl and mixing together the green onions and the PB2.
2. Then take out a plate and heat up the tortillas inside of the microwave for about 20 seconds.
3. Place the dressing on top of the tortilla and then add in the vegetables and chicken. Wrap up the tortilla and then enjoy.

Pita Bread Pizza – 9 SmartPoints®

Ingredients:

2 tsp. Parmesan cheese
Pinch of pizza seasoning
10 chopped black olives
½ c. mozzarella cheese
¼ c. mushrooms, sliced
¼ c. green pepper
1 pita bread
¼ c. pizza sauce

Directions:

1. Lay out the pita bread and put the pizza sauce all over it. Top this with the seasoning, mozzarella, parmesan cheese, and vegetables.
2. Spray this with a bit of cooking spray and then place it on a baking pan. Turn on the oven to broil.
3. Put the pita into the oven and let it broil in the oven for 2 minutes to let the cheese melt. Take it out of the oven and let it cool down for a bit before serving.

Bacon & Potato Soup – 4 SmartPoints®

Ingredients:

1 c. water
6 Tbsp. bacon bits
1 pack of gravy
1 c. skim milk
32 oz. hash browns, non-fat
3 cans chicken broth

Directions:

1. Bring out a pot and coat it with some cooking spray. Heat it up and then add in the hash browns.
2. After a few minutes, add in the chicken broth and bring this to a boil before lowering the heat and letting this come to a simmer.

3. While the hash browns are heating up, take out another bowl and mix together the gravy mix, water, and milk.
4. Pour this mixture in with the cooked potatoes and then add in the bacon bits. Cook this for a little bit longer to allow it time to thicken. Season with some salt and then serve.

Roast Beef with Veggies – 8 SmartPoints®

Ingredients:

14 oz. diced tomatoes
1 pack onion soup mix
4 carrots, chunked
1 onion, quartered
2 roast beef
2 lbs. wedged potatoes

Directions:

1. Place the roast into your slow cooker and then top it with the onion soup mix.
2. When that is organized, add in the carrots, onion, and potatoes and then top with the tomatoes.
3. Place the cover onto the slow cooker and let this cook on a low setting for about 7 hours.

Mushroom Steak – 5 SmartPoints®

Ingredients:

2 tsp. Worcestershire sauce
Parsley
2 Tbsp. flour
2 Tbsp. tomato paste
1/8 tsp. pepper
8 oz. sliced mushrooms
2 c. beef broth
¼ tsp. salt
1 egg
1 egg white
1 lb. ground turkey
½ c. bread crumbs
1 ½ tsp. cooking oil
¾ c. onions, minced
½ tsp. mustard powder
¼ c. water
1 tsp. red wine vinegar

Directions:

1. Take out a skillet and cook the oil and the onions together for about 5 minutes.
2. Bring out a bowl and mix together the black pepper, salt, egg, egg white, ground turkey, bread crumbs, half of the cooked onions, ¼ cup of the beef broth, and the ground beef.
3. When this is all combined, use our hands to form these into 8 patties. Add into the skillet and cook on each side to brown.

4. Add the pepper, salt, and mushrooms into the skillet and cook for another 3 minutes. Then add the patties back inside.
5. While that is cooking, mix together the broth and the flour. Then add in the Worcestershire sauce, mustard powder, vinegar, water, tomato paste, and the rest of the onions.
6. Pour this sauce over the meat and mushrooms in the skillet. Serve it warm.

Cheese and Tuna Sandwich – 10 SmartPoints®

Ingredients:

1 sliced tomato
½ c. cheddar cheese
1 ½ Tbsp. butter
2 Tbsp. spicy brown mustard
1 ½ Tbsp. pickle relish
4 slices bread
5 oz. can tuna
1 ½ Tbsp. mayo

Directions:

1. Bring out a bowl and combine together the pickle relish, drained tuna, and the mayo.
2. Lay out the bread and spread out some butter on one of the slices and then mustard on the other.

3. Put the cheese, tomato, and tuna on the side with the mustard and then place the other two slices on top to make our sandwich.
4. Place these both into a pan and then cover and cook for 3 minutes on both sides. Cut in half and then enjoy!

Cola Chicken – 5 SmartPoints®

Ingredients:

1 can of diet cola
½ c. onion, chopped
4 chicken breasts, skinless
1 c. ketchup

Directions:

1. Bring out a skillet to start this recipe and combine the cola and the ketchup inside.
2. After a few minutes, add in the chicken and the onions and stir it all around. Bring this to a boil before placing the cover on top and reducing the heat.
3. Simmer the whole meal together for about 45 minutes so that the chicken has time to marinate before serving.

Beef Chili – 4 SmartPoints®

Ingredients:
2 Tbsp. tomato paste
Pepper
1 chopped sweet onion
¼ c. diced green chilies
28 oz. tomatoes in a can
15 oz. red kidney beans,
2 Tbsp. chili powder
2 tsp. cumin
1 diced red bell pepper
1 diced green bell pepper
1 lb. ground turkey or beef
1 Tbsp. minced garlic

Directions:
1. To start this recipe, bring out a skillet and brown the ground beef together with the garlic. When these are done cooking, take the fat out of the skillet and then add in the bell peppers.
2. Cook this for 5 minutes so that the peppers can get nice and soft. Now add in the chili powder and cumin and cook for a few more minutes.
3. Bring out a slow cooker and add in the meat mixture, tomato paste, chilies, onion, tomatoes, and kidney beans inside.
4. Put the lid on top of the slow cooker and let this cook for about 5 hours. When you are ready to serve, season with some black pepper and serve.

Vegetable Quesadilla – 9 SmartPoints®

Ingredients:
Cooking spray
¼ c. shredded cheddar cheese
¼ c. shredded mozzarella cheese
Salt
2 wheat flour tortillas
1 dash cayenne pepper
Pepper
1 Tbsp. red bell pepper, diced
1 tsp. soy sauce
1/3 c. shredded carrot
1/3 c. broccoli, chopped
½ Tbsp. canola oil
½ c. mushrooms, sliced

Directions:
1. To start this recipe, bring out a pan and cook up the vegetables inside for 7 minutes to make it nice and soft. Season with the salt, soy sauce, and the peppers.
2. When the vegetables are all done cooking place them into the bowl.
3. Clean out the pan if needed and place one of the tortillas inside. Top with half the cheese, some vegetables, and then the remainder of the cheese. Place the second tortilla on top.
4. Heat this for about 2 minutes to make it nice and warm. After that time, turn the quesadilla over and let it cook for another minute before serving.

Baked Chicken – 10 SmartPoints®

Ingredients:

2 Tbsp. Worcestershire sauce
2 tsp. dry mustard
3 Tbsp. brown sugar
2 Tbsp. vinegar
4 chicken breasts
½ c. ketchup

Directions:

1. Turn on the oven and let it heat up to 350 degrees.
2. While the oven is heating up, place the chicken into the baking dish and then add in the ketchup, vinegar, brown sugar, dry mustard, and Worcestershire sauce all around the chicken.
3. Place these into the oven and bake the meal for 40 minutes. Allow some time to cool down before serving.

Chicken and Dumplings – 9 SmartPoints®

Ingredients:
Tortillas
Pepper
Salt
½ Tbsp. celery salt

3 c. chicken breast, chopped
2 cans chicken broth
1 can cream of chicken soup

Directions:
1. Take out a pan and add together the chicken breast, cream of chicken soup, and chicken broth. Sprinkle in the seasonings.
2. Add the tortillas one at a time. Reduce the heat and let it simmer for 25 minutes.

Conclusion

Weight Watchers is one of the best diet pans that you can choose to go on. It is easy to follow and you are going to love how much good food you are able to enjoy while losing weight. While some of the other diet plans that you may have tried in the past focused too much on telling you a long list of foods that you weren't allowed to eat, Weight Watchers allows you to live life and eat good foods all at the same time.

Going on a diet should be something that you can do for a lifetime, not something that you get disappointed with because it is too hard to maintain for the long term. Weight Watchers will be able to help you to do all of this, even if you have tried and failed with other diets in the past.

Inside this guidebook, you will get the information that you need in order to get started with the Weight Watchers plan. We offer a bit of information to get you started and then work on a 30-day meal plan, complete with all of the recipes that you need in order to get the best results. You aren't going to believe how tasty and fulfilling some of these meals can be, but they will help you to lose weight and feel great!

So take a look through this guidebook and find out just how easy and tasty the Weight Watchers diet can be!

Michael Smith

Preview of my next book:

Weight Watchers Instant Pot Cookbook

Benefits of Using Instant Pot

Even though pressure cookers in general have been around for many years, there are still many people who don't use them because they don't realize the benefits that they hold. The reality is that there are many different benefits to using a pressure cooker and Instant Pot specifically, and while we only have enough space to cover a handful of them here, we will go over the most valuable ones.

BENEFIT #1: YOUR FOOD WILL PRESERVE ALMOST ALL NUTRITIONAL VALUE

We've touched on this one already, but your food will preserve far more of its nutritional value when cooked in an Instant Pot (or any pressure cooker for that matter) versus other cooking methods. The main reason why is because other cooking methods take longer to cook the food, and the longer that foods are being cooked, then the more vitamins and nutrients will be eliminated.

Pressure cooking cooks foods in less time and in less liquid. And since the liquid itself is being boiled, this will only naturally leave the food with more nutrients. It should be noted as well that less cooking time doesn't just preserve more of the nutritional value of the food, but it also preserves more of the taste as well.

BENEFIT #2: YOU WILL SAVE ENERGY

Pressure cookers in general will allow you to save on energy because it's simply a more efficient cooking method than other cooking processes. For one thing, you can cook your food entirely in one pot with one burner. You don't need to use any other pots and pans or cooking surfaces. And furthermore, there's that less cooking time, which furthermore reduces energy.

There's no denying that our electric bills aren't always generous. That's why it's wise to always be seeking ways to reduce energy and your consumption of electricity in order to decrease the amount of money that you pay each month in bills.

BENEFIT #3: YOU'LL SAVE TIME

Again, here's that overall reduced cooking time kicking in as well. While the actual cooking time varies by the meal or food, there are some foods that will be able to have a 70% less cooking time in a pressure cooker than if there were cooked in another method such as frying, baking, or grilling. This makes Instant Pot and pressure cooking in general a very practical method for cooking and enables you to get food more quickly on the table.

You may have thought that you would never be able to whip up a full meal in mere minutes, but with a pressure cooker it's possible. All you have to do is simply throw all of the ingredients into the pressure cooker, and then cook it for as long as the directions say to. Less time spent cooking in the kitchen gives you more time to spend doing other things in the evening such as relaxing, spending time with the family, or enjoying your favorite hobbies.

BENEFIT #4: YOU CAN ALSO PRESERVE FOOD

There's a reason why pressure cookers are popular with survivalists or those who like to can their food for the long term. As long as you have a larger pressure cooker, you can seal up meats or vegetables inside jars or cans and then place them into the pressure cooker. Assuming your pressure cooker is capable of developing pressure up to 15 PSI, you can then cook the food in the can or jar and then store it at ideal room temperatures for the long term. Many of the larger models of pressure canners will sell with a separate set of instructions that are specifically on how to can foods. In order to ensure that your food is preserve safely, you must follow these instructions very carefully.

These are the primary benefits to using a pressure cooker in general. Instant Pot specifically is easily the most technologically advanced and most efficient type of pressure cooker that is sold on the marketplace today. One reason why is because it serves a multitude of different functions. For example, the latest models of Instant Pot combine pressure cooking, slow cooking, steaming, a sauté pan, yogurt maker, and a porridge maker all in the same device at once.

So in addition to the general benefits of pressure cooking that we have just talked about, you should also keep these benefits in mind that are unique to Instant Pot specifically, the first of which is obviously versatility. If you wanted to, you could use Instant Pot as your sole cooking device in your kitchen. This permits you to clean up your kitchen by removing a lot of the clutter that exists in it and instead predominately using your Instant Pot. And just like pressure cookers in general, Instant Pot is very energy efficient, and preserves all of the nutrients and taste of the food that you are preparing.

Now that we have learned about how to use Instant Pot and the benefits of doing so and pressure cooking in general, for the rest of this e-book we're going to go over the top recommended recipes that you can cook in your Instant Pot machine. We'll be covering recipes for breakfast, lunch, dinner, dessert, and snack and appetizers in that order.

What you need to do now is pull out a notepad and a writing utensil, and as you read down through this list of recipes, take a note of the ones that seem the most appealing to you. This way it will be easier for you to find them for when you decide to use your Instant Pot machine for the first time, and it also makes it easier for gathering the necessary ingredients that you will need as well.

Keep in mind that you'll never truly know whether you like or dislike a recipe before you actually try that, so have an open mind about each of these recipes and think about what you believe you and your family will enjoy the most.

1. 5 Easy Steps to Use Electric Pressure Cooker for making any food:

1. Fill electric pressure cooker pot with ingredients, along with 1 ½ cups of cooking liquid like water or broth. If the ingredients are beans and grains fill pot half full, while fill pot two-third full for the other ingredients. Now switch on electric pressure cooker.
2. Manually or automatically close lid and double check it with pressure indicator. If cooker is lock correctly, the indicator will lift.

3. Punch in cooking time or choose from built-in cooking setting.
4. Pressure will build up in cooker, this usually takes 10-15 minutes and this is followed by pressure cooking of food. The timer will display the time.
5. Upon finished pressure cooking, release pressure. Choose natural release or quick release. Don't open cooker until pressure is release completely and pressure indicator drop down.

Begin with your electric pressure cooking lessons with the following 30 easy and detailed recipes. Each recipe will teach you skills that will help you pressure cooking any conventional recipe. The cookbook contains three recipe sections: breakfast, lunches and dinners. Take a leap and try cooking in an electric pressure cooker.

That is enough information for the cooker, now it is time to make some delicious food we all love to eat with the following recipes.

Remembers, anyone can cook

Photo are only for display purpose and may belong to respective owners

Maple Smoked Brisket and Carrot

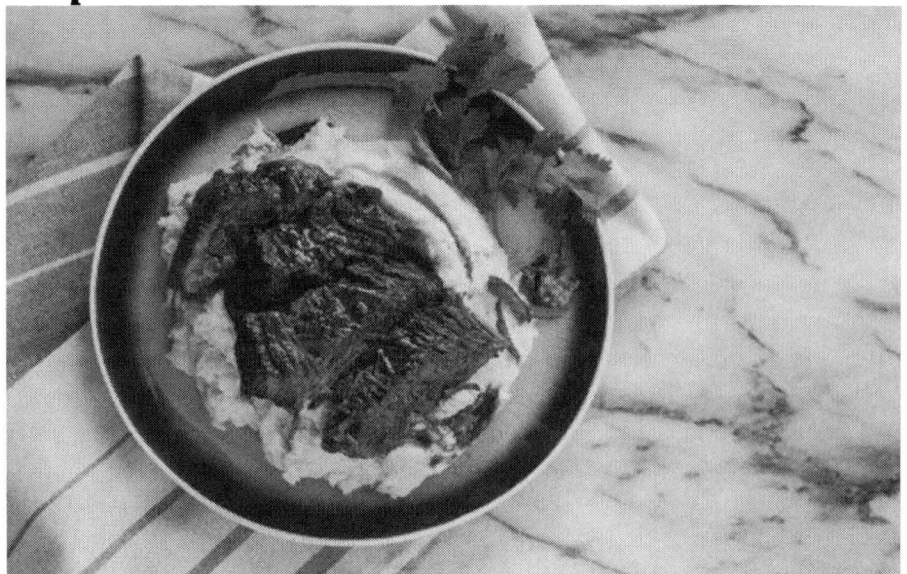

Preparation time: 30 minutes
Cooking Time: 59 minutes
Servings: 7
6 Points
Pressure: High
Ingredients Main Dish
- 2 Kgs beef brisket
- 2Tablespoons Olive oil.
- 2 Tablespoons coconut sugar
- 2 Tablespoons smoked sea salt
- 2 Tablespoons black pepper
- 1 Tablespoon mustard powder
- 1 Tablespoon onion powder
- I Tablespoon smoked paprika
- 2 Cups chicken stock.
- 1 Tablespoon liquid smoke
- 3 fresh thyme sprigs

Side Dish

* 1/2 Cup sour cream
* 2 Tablespoons white wine vinegar
* 1/2 Tablespoon ground cumin
* 1 Tablespoon kosher salt and black pepper respectively
* 3/4 Pound large carrots, peeled
* 2 Granny Smith apples, halved and cored
* 1/2 Cup golden raisins
* 1/4 Cup chopped cilantro

Directions Main Course:
* Refrigerate the brisket for 20 minutes before you cook it. Dry using kitchen paper towels
* Combine the coconut sugar, pepper, smoked sea salt, onion powder, mustard powder, and the smoked paprika.
* Switch on the pressure cooker and adjust to sauté. Leave it to heat for 2 minutes.
* Add 1 tablespoon of Olive oil and add the brisket. Allow it brown on both sides careful not to burn it.
* Add the chicken stock, thyme and liquid smoke to the pressure cooker.
* Adjust to cooker setting to manual and leave for 50 minutes.
* Allow the cooker to release the pressure naturally.
* Remove the meat and cover with a foil.
* The remnants in the cooker can make an excellent sauce. If you want, you can adjust the cooker into sauté and continue boiling for 5 minutes to thicken the broth. (Don't cover)

Directions Side Dish (Takes less than 2 minutes)

* In a mixing bowl, add yoghurt, cumin, vinegar, 1/2 Tablespoon salt, and 1/4 Tablespoon pepper.
* Grate the carrots and apples in a food processor.
* Mix in the bowl the apples, raisins, carrots, cilantro, and carrots to the sour cream and combine.
* Indulge yourself with the brisket.

Tip: You can skip the liquid smoke but you'll get faint smoke flavor.

I've have also found out that increasing or decreasing your meat size by 1 lb. You will require about a 20 minute change in cooking time.

Steamed Artichokes
Servings: About 4
Cooking Time: 7 minutes
Total Time: 20 minutes
2 Points

Whether you enjoy artichokes cooked and on their own or with a dipping sauce, this recipe gives you both, although the recipe is much healthier when you choose to eat the artichokes by themselves.

INGREDIENTS

2 artichokes of medium size (or you can use various sizes, refer to the steam instructions for the different sizes of artichokes)

1 cup of water
1 lemon cut in half
2 tablespoons of mayonnaise
1 teaspoon of Dijon mustard

1 pinch of paprika

Depending on size, you can steam pieces in increments of 5 minutes. For instance, 5 for a small piece, 10 for medium, and 15 for large.

DIRECTIONS

1. Your artichokes need to be cleaned up with kitchen spears. Cut off any of the spiny edges and woody pieces. Trim off any spines of the surrounding leaves. If there are any damaged leaves, remove them.
2. Wash the artichokes off in water. You can use your lemon slices to wipe any edges that you cut. This will keep them from oxidizing. You can give the artichokes a stable base to rest on during the cooking process by slicing the stems off and creating a flat surface.

3. Place the steamer rack in your instant pot and then pour in the water. Place the artichokes on the rack facing upwards. You can spritz any remaining lemon juice over the artichokes for an added taste during the cooking process.

4. Close the lid of the instant pot and lock. Then, you will cook the artichokes for ten minutes on high pressure.

5. After the cooking process is complete, you should use the natural release process in order to release the pressure from your instant pot.

6. The doneness of the artichokes can be checked by doing a taste test. Take one of the leaves and check the level of softness. If your artichokes are too firm for your taste, you can cook them for a few more minutes. Use the normal release method once the cooking time is done.

7. Once your artichokes are done cooking, you can make a dipping mix to go with them. Mix together the mayonnaise with the Dijon mustard and sprinkle paprika over the mixture. Serve your artichokes fresh and warm.

Made in the USA
San Bernardino, CA
26 October 2018